ACCESS TO
MEDICAL KNOWLEDGE

Libraries, Digitization, and the Public Good

FRANCES K. GROEN

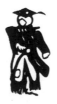

THE SCARECROW PRESS, INC.
Lanham, Maryland • Toronto • Plymouth, UK
2007

SCARECROW PRESS, INC.

Published in the United States of America
by Scarecrow Press, Inc.
A wholly owned subsidiary of
The Rowman & Littlefield Publishing Group, Inc.
4501 Forbes Boulevard, Suite 200, Lanham, Maryland 20706
www.scarecrowpress.com

Estover Road
Plymouth PL6 7PY
United Kingdom

British Library Cataloguing in Publication Information Available

Library of Congress Cataloging-in-Publication Data

Groen, Frances K.
  Access to medical knowledge : libraries, digitization, and the public good /
Frances K. Groen.
     p. ; cm.
  Includes bibliographical references and index.
  ISBN-13: 978-0-8108-5272-3 (pbk. : alk. paper)
  ISBN-10: 0-8108-5272-1 (pbk. : alk. paper)
   1. Medical informatics—Moral and ethical aspects. 2. Medical libraries—Moral
and ethical aspects. 3. Medical librarians—Moral and ethical aspects. 4.
Information technology—Moral and ethical aspects. I. Title.
  [DNLM: 1. Access to Information—ethics. 2. Libraries, Medical—ethics. 3.
History, 19th Century. 4. History, 20th Century. 5. Information Management—
methods. 6. Internet. 7. Libraries, Medical—history. Z 675.M4 G874a 2007]

R858.G76 2007
610.285—dc22   2006020465

To the memory of my parents,
Johanna and Milton.

CONTENTS

PART IV: IS THERE A BETTER WAY?

PREFACE

This book was written as an attempt to understand why librarians, whether working in the health care environment or in the academic milieu, make the choices and develop the services that they do. Are they guided by principles or values within a conceptual framework, or are they merely responding opportunistically to a variety of influences—institutional, social, technical, and political? During the forty-plus years of my professional practice, my work has not left me with an abundance of time for reflection on my profession and the values upon which it is built. During my career, I moved around a good deal in the earlier stages, both geographically and intellectually . . . from a large Canadian academic library, where I found my first professional appointment, to a large medical library in the United States and then to another large academic library, another large medical library, then back to Canada, first in a medical library and then in my final professional appointment back in the academic library milieu. I had also flirted with the history and philosophy of science when I did graduate work in this area. This accounts, perhaps, for my lifelong interest in the history of libraries and for my particular interest in the history of medicine, although I shall always remain an amateur in these areas. It is also the reason that this work has raked the historical coals of the development of medical librarianship. For a highly professional treatment of this subject the reader is referred to the work of historian Jennifer Connor and her sprightly monograph, *Guardians of Medical Knowledge: The Genesis of the Medical Library Association*.

The issue of values both personal and professional is a matter of increasing interest in the world today. Was there a recognizable past in medical libraries that continued to enrich and inform present practice? To answer this question, I needed to look at libraries before and after the Internet changed the world. Since I had spent more than a quarter of a century of my professional life in medical libraries in Canada and the United States, the medical library seemed a good place to start to explore this question. Identifying evidence of shared professional values remained a primary concern throughout the writing. Using the medical library literature that extended over more than a century, I was able to identify three professional values—providing access to the medical literature for all who require it, empowering and educating library users, and preserving the wisdom of the past. The *Journal of the Medical Library Association* acts in some ways as the journal of record for the profession, and its complete and public availability in PubMed Central, the U.S. National Library of Medicine's repository, made my task much simpler. This digital archive provides a strong example of careful digitization and the virtue of open access, an issue of concern in the Internet era that is explored in the later part of this book.

The reader will notice that both the Medical Library Association headquartered in Chicago and the U.S. National Library of Medicine play a large role in this book. This is as it should be. The Medical Library Association is the largest and oldest organization serving medical librarians worldwide. It has membership in many parts of the world, and four of its presidents have been Canadian. The U.S. National Library of Medicine has produced the indexes, databases, and other resources that are used worldwide, and its programs and policies have facilitated access to health information globally. At the same time, I have attempted to remind the reader of some of the initiatives, particularly in other parts of the English-speaking world, outside of the United States, especially in Canada.

International medical librarianship and global access to the medical literature has been a lifelong interest and commitment for me. Through generous institution support, I have had the opportunity to participate in the six international congresses on medical libraries held between 1980 and 2005. In organizing this book, I had originally intended to develop a chapter that would be devoted to this topic. However, as the writing progressed, it became clear that it would be better to integrate international medical librarianship into the context of the times in which these congresses were held. More work needs to be done on this topic, and if I were to do it, it would take the form of a book on issues in global access to the literature of medicine.

I have drawn heavily upon my own involvement in medical libraries and in the work of various associations with which I have worked throughout my career, beginning in the 1960s. The notes, reports, memos, proceedings, and minutes from my work with various associations that have cluttered my home and my office have finally justified their retention. These resources needed to be validated by the official print and archival record, cited in the notes for the chapters, and included in the final bibliography. I want to thank the executive director of the Medical Library Association, Carla Funk, for permission to quote from work published in their journal; Blackwell publishing, Oxford, the publisher of *Health Libraries Review*, for allowing me to reproduce material from an article originally published in that journal on the Canadian National Site Licensing initiative; and the Management Committee on the McGill Libraries journal, *Fontanus*, for its permission as well.

Writing a book is a matter of selecting material to include, and therefore, choosing what not to discuss. This was for me one of the most difficult tasks. No two individuals will agree on what or whom to include in a history that covers more than one hundred years. There are many individuals who have made outstanding contributions to the advancement of medical libraries whose names are not mentioned nor their work recognized in this book. This omission is in no sense a measure of my regard for their enduring value to the profession. I hope that they will recognize that their omission from my little book is not a reflection on my respect for their work.

The complete and comprehensive change that the Internet brought about in medical libraries required a quite different approach to the organization of material in the final chapters of this work. In the first two sections, the overall organization is chronological, but due to the accelerated speed of recent developments, this approach did not seem to fit the material. The book begins with the identification of the three core values of medical librarians and then identifies how these values are reflected over time in the work of medical librarians—in war and in peace, in prosperity and austerity. When the Internet arrived in the medical library, this essentially chronological approach was no longer valid for a variety of reasons. In the Internet era, the time frame is very short, changes are very rapid, and they are likewise fundamental. Instead, a topical approach was chosen, looking at the core value of providing access to information in relation to clinical information and consumer health information. The economic challenge of providing access to medical and scientific information is reviewed, and some of the alternatives in the age of the Internet are explored. In addressing the costs of providing access to the scholarly record, librarians are seen to make common cause with researchers, administrators, and teachers in the interests of promoting access to information. I discuss the revolution in medical and scientific communication brought about by the Internet, which, while it involves and profoundly affects the medical library in all its functions, is of course a process that transcends the library. A word of caution—the period covered ends in early 2006, and the reader will need to go further than this to see how certain debates will resolve, if they ever do.

This is my opportunity to express my gratitude to the Harold Crabtree Foundation for its generous support of my project. Its grant enabled me to maintain my knowledge through visits with colleagues and participation in meetings during my sabbatical leave, tracking the very most recent developments. This grant has also enabled me to continue my professional involvement. To Sandra Crabtree and her board goes my enduring gratitude for their generous support. The Harold Crabtree Foundation supported libraries at McGill throughout my years there, and I hope that this work will justify this investment in a librarian.

My husband, Jean-Claude Guédon, has been at my side during my writing. His deep knowledge of the history of science and of scientific communication, along with his expertise in electronic scholar publishing, informed my understanding as I worked. Numerous discussions, e-mails with monumental attachments, and lovely dinners cheered me on when I felt unequal to my task. In particular, Jean-Claude is a strong participant in the open-access initiative, having participated in the Budapest and Berlin meetings. There is no doubt that his thinking has been formative for a number of people, and it would be false to pretend that it has not influenced my position on the open-access initiative.

Introduction

LIBRARIES AS A PUBLIC GOOD—WHY?

In many parts of the world, the idea of the library occupies a privileged position in the public lexicon of values. This is not to say that the library is first to benefit from the public purse of financial support. But the idea of the library, so integrally linked with the idea of literacy and an open society, has managed, quite justifiably, to secure an iconic significance in society at large.

One of my earliest memories as a small child growing up in southern Ontario was going to the local public library with my mother. She took my child's hand firmly in her protective grasp as we marched up the impressive set of stairs leading to these magnificent, wooden double doors of that Carnegie grant library. We entered a large, domed foyer through which we slipped as silently as possible, to emerge in the vast, radiating stacks of the library. This was a precious place, to both adult and child. As an immigrant to Canada, my mother had arrived, not knowing a word of English. But she had learned to love reading in her native Dutch, in her country of birth, and she had found her way to the library in her new home. And she learned English as her second language, through a variety of teachers from Zane Grey to Leo Tolstoy. I was shocked by the beauty and the reverence of that place, smiling people behind desks, with stamp pads in red and black, old men from whose hands newspapers on long wooden rods would slip as the afternoon progressed.

In my working high school days—I believe I was fourteen at the time—I managed to find temporary work at this same library during the summer and after school. My mind went into fantasy as I imagined myself a "keeper of books," not knowing that the "Keeper of Books" was a distinguished title at Oxford University Library. At the same time, and with a sense of commitment equal to my mother's zeal for reading, my father assumed responsibility for bringing me home from the library when it closed in the evening. But he never climbed the impressive staircase or crossed the marble rotunda, preferring to wait outside until I emerged after the library closed. For him too, the library had great iconic value, but it was also a place of intimidation, since he had never achieved literacy.

Libraries are synonymous with literacy, but in today's world, the concept of literacy has become far more varied. It has broadened to include a number of conceptual skills in numeracy and arithmetic. But in a civil society it has taken on even greater meaning, as it gives the power to the people. In a quite remarkable 1990 address to the Saskatchewan Library Association that remains relevant fifteen years later, Stephen Lewis, former Canadian ambassador to the United States and special adviser to the United Nations on Africa, gave us a powerfully comprehensive definition of contemporary literacy.

> The most profound, far reaching and significant impact of literacy on people's lives is its empowering potential. To be literate is to become liberated from the constraints of dependency. To be literate is to gain a voice and to participate meaningfully and assertively in the decisions that affect people's lives. To be literate is to become politically conscious, critically aware and to de-mystify social reality. Literacy enables people to read one's own word and to write history. Literacy makes people aware of their basic human rights. Literacy enables people to have a greater degree of control over their own lives. Literacy helps people to become self-reliant and to resist exploitation and repression. Literacy provides access to written knowledge and knowledge is power.[1]

Today's world is concerned with the digital divide and computer literacy, yet the need of yesterday's world for simple and powerful literacy has yet to be fully satisfied. This is analogous to librarians focusing on the problem of digital preservation while the full magnitude of the problem of print preservation has yet to be addressed. Creativity and technology have given us a new world that exists contemporaneously with the legacy of the past. The library at the beginning of the twenty-first century is the theater and the laboratory in which the reconciliation of past and future must be developed. Librarians must acquire and make available collections to support a literate public, depending on resources and the nature and mission of the library. Even in the most specialized libraries, opportunities will exist to act in the public good and to promote a literate, knowledgeable society. A particularly strong case for acting in the public good can be argued for all libraries and institutions supported by public funds. A proactive role for the library is needed, both to promote the public good and to ensure a strong, viable position for the library in the contemporary cultural and educational scene. Lectures, public events, and publications promote the library, and at the same time sponsor a deep understanding of the library as a source of knowledge regarding both past and present. Each kind of library will have a unique set of opportunities to support the public good.

In the world of libraries, promotion of literacy and the significance of the library are being both enhanced and threatened by information technology. Nothing can substitute for the power of the written word and the world of ideas. In the print world, reading tended to favor commentary, analysis, and even meditation; reading in the computer age seems to foster a sort of "PowerPoint" approach to knowledge. Today's universities are faced with students who never knew a world without computers. At the same time, the problems of escalating costs, including the very high financial demands of information and communications technologies, are pushing administrators to see genuine solutions in technology applications. The electronic classroom and online instruction have become panaceas for both the improvement of student learning and cost effectiveness. In this environment, librarians have a valuable, leading role to play in sustaining literacy and the iconic values of the library; as citizens they have a potentially powerful voice in enforcing the drain of the university on the public purse, and the strongest of all their arguments will be the demonstration of the fact that the library serves a public good.

AN OPPORTUNITY: THE WORLD
SUMMIT ON THE INFORMATION SOCIETY

In his message to the World Summit on the Information Society (WSIS), United Nations Secretary-General Kofi Annan spoke of a world in which information is omnipresent, through newspapers, radio, television, and the Internet.[2] The secretary-general describes our world as one "in which information is transforming the ways in which we live, learn, work and relate; and in which information is indispensable—for health, agriculture, education and trade, and for cultivating the engaged and learned citizenry that is essential for democracy to work."[3] He continues, emphasizing the challenge of "what to do with the masses of information and knowledge increasingly at our disposal."[4] It is difficult not to wonder why, in this world where literacy is essential to a democratic society, and where "masses" of information cry out for an organizing principle in order to make them functional, Mr. Annan neglected the role that the library can play in literacy and in organizing information for use. Mr. Annan speaks with compassion for the world's people who, through poverty and illiteracy, have remained untouched by the information revolution. Libraries have a role to play in solving problems of access and literacy. Could not libraries contribute to solving problems of access, freedom, and privacy? Do not libraries have a role to play in envisioning, as he describes, "a shared vision of an information society that empowers and benefits all people"?

The international community of libraries became concerned to create an opportunity for librarians to play an active role in this summit. Representation from numerous groups—scientists, the private sector, governments, civil society groups, the media, and the press were partnering, and the importance of this event was not lost on librarians. As a result, under the sponsorship of the International Federation of Library Associations and Institutions, a preconference summit was organized to prepare for the forthcoming WSIS meeting.

Discussions resulted in a strong statement of the value of libraries in promoting a global information commons, a vision of "an inclusive Information Society in which everyone can create, access, use and share information and knowledge and which is based on the fundamental right of human beings to both access and express information without restriction."[5] The statement recognizes the role of the library in enabling access past political boundaries and over time to create a global information resource and a community of users able to benefit from the revolution in information technology. It recognizes, too, that libraries have already invested heavily in information infrastructure and electronic information resources, and that these significant investments can and should play a role in the world information society.

From small public libraries in the pre-automation era, to a world summit on information, the library plays a role in sustaining the public good through promoting literate citizens and providing access to information. The iconic value of the library as well as the proactive role played by librarians provide strong support for the promotion of the public good.

NOTES

1. Stephen Lewis, "The Struggle for Literacy Abroad and at Home," from *The International Task Force on Literacy Newsletter*, 1990, in *Survival of the Imagination: The Mary Donaldson Memorial Lectures*, ed. Brett Baker and Peter Resch (Regina, SK: Coteau Books, 1993), 283.

2. Kofi Annan, "WSIS: Connecting the World Summit on the Information Society," First Phase: Geneva December 10–12, 2003, 1.

3. Annan, "WSIS: Connecting the World," 1.

4. Annan, "WSIS: Connecting the World," 1.

5. IFLANET, "Promoting the Global Information Commons," IFLA response to the WSIS Declaration, http://www.IFLA.ORG/iii/WSIS060604 .html (accessed September 15, 2004).

I

LIBRARIANS AND THEIR VALUES

1

LIBRARIANS, VALUES, AND
THE PUBLIC GOOD

This book is about the work of medical librarians in support of the idea of the public good. It is also about public goods and the importance of viewing information as "public goods" in the way public education and highways are public goods. Providing access to information to all who need to use it is one of three core values of the library profession; the other two values that are at the heart of the practice of librarianship are the promotion of literacy and the preservation of the accumulated wisdom of the past. It can be argued that all librarians share an appreciation of these values regardless of the type of library in which they practice their profession. The expression of these shared values forms the tie that binds members of the profession together. But the particular way in which these core values are interpreted in medical libraries is what creates medical librarianship as a distinct profession. These values are perennial, and have been demonstrated by medical librarians since the founding of their profession, as seen in the review of the history of medical libraries that forms a part of this book.

New challenges have arisen in the provision of access to information, ones that are both positive and negative, as information became increasingly commodified in the electronic era. Acting in the public good to provide access to information to all who need it is threatened when access is limited to only those who are able to pay for it. Public goods have been defined as "consumer goods that, when made available to anyone, can be made available to others at no additional cost."[1] Public goods exist for the public good, and it can be argued that medical information can be considered as a form of public goods. If this definition of goods as usable by ever increasing numbers of individuals at no additional cost is applied to information, a rethinking of the costs and availability of certain kinds of information, including medical information, becomes necessary. In electronic form, the journal may be regarded as public goods, since it may be distributed to all who wish to read it at no additional cost. This definition of public goods is not sufficiently complete to resolve the dilemma of public information in the digital age. What is necessary is a rethinking of the information economy. Only when information is accepted both as a public good and as public goods can librarians provide the necessary information to those who need to use it.

The past two decades have seen intense political debate over what is considered public and private. Privatization has become a dominant ideology in many developed countries, and the concepts of "public good" and "public goods" are being redefined as this book is being written. The Millennium Road Map of the United Nations identifies ten global goals,[2] three of which have particular relevance to the role of medical librarians and the public good:

1. dignity for all people, including access to basic education and health care
2. global public health, particularly communicable disease control
3. concerted management of knowledge, including worldwide respect for intellectual property rights

These three goals are deeply grounded in health care and health information. Good health care delivery requires access to the best and most recent knowledge contained in the published medical literature. Global public health requires that citizens are educated and become knowledgeable in order to participate in the maintenance of their personal health. And intellectual property management requires a judicious balance by librarians between the rights of consumers and of creators.

A PROFESSION IN TRANSITION

Modern librarianship, whether practiced in a public, university, medical, or business setting, is the effort of educated librarians and information professionals who share a commitment to the values, services, and techniques of the profession. The delivery of information services and the technical infrastructure required to support these services are the basis for core curriculum development in the graduate programs of library and information studies. However, the teaching of the values of the profession is less well developed. Perhaps the library curriculum in universities is already overextended and leaves little space for the study of a topic, the mastery of which does not result in a set of skills necessary to obtain that first professional appointment. Perhaps educators feel that values are inculcated in the practice of the profession, rather than in the classroom. Recently, however, there has been a renewal of interest in the values underlying the profession of librarianship, especially evident in the writing of Michael Gorman.[3]

Gorman explains the renewal of interest in the values of the profession as the result of the great changes that the library profession, like society at large, is undergoing and the disconnect between library educators and library practitioners. The extraordinary impact of information and communications technologies (ICT) on the profession and on library budgets has raised fundamental questions about the practice of librarianship as well. ICT has brought transformative change to libraries, change that is both incremental and revolutionary. Librarians who enter the profession today may never work in a library. Even if they do manage to find positions in established libraries, they may never work with books. The "virtual library" is more real to many librarians than the library with walls. These new-generation librarians have never known a world without computers and are likely to have written their student essays using Google.

If further evidence of the transformation of the library profession is necessary, consider the sometimes desperate efforts to find new and possibly more attractive ways of naming the professional librarian. "Cyberians," "knowledge navigators," "information professionals," "digital librarians," are just a few of the new labels that are being used. This is perhaps as it should be in a period of profound restructuring. However, the renaming of the practitioner and acquisition of a set of skills, no matter how sophisticated, are not sufficient to sustain a profession in a period of profound transformation. Librarians understand this and have articulated their values through an examination of their professional belief system and in their willingness to reflect in a meaningful way on why they make certain choices in the daily practice of their profession. Absorbed in a profession that is both highly pragmatic and extremely process oriented, a librarian may develop only gradually these values that inform practice. However these values are developed, whether in the acquisition of the professional credential or on the job, they provide the conceptual framework for the practice of the profession. These values are explored conceptually in this chapter; they guide the historical review of medical libraries in part 2 of this book; and recur in the final section on medical libraries in the age of the Internet, particularly with respect to discussions around public access to medical information.

Librarians in general have become synonymous with three fundamental values that support a belief in access to information, universal literacy, and preservation of cultural heritage. These values are also enshrined as characteristics of liberal democratic societies, in both the print and electronic age of libraries. Two of these values—access to information and universal literacy—are also attributes of an open society and an informed and responsible citizenry. Librarians have nurtured these values over time and have been challenged by social forces that have viewed information as a commodity that can be bought and sold, access to which is determined by the reader/consumer's ability to pay.

LIBRARIES AND ACCESS TO INFORMATION IN THE PUBLIC GOOD

If information is viewed as a commodity, it is inevitable that access to this commodity will be limited. A variety of ways exists to limit this commodity; it is not difficult to think of them. The number of libraries can be reduced, their budgets can be cut, the libraries might be required to charge users to access their resources, and many other possible controls designed to provide access to information only to those who are able and willing to pay for it. This scenario will develop if information is viewed as a product that is produced and sold. Its availability is limited, as is any commodity, since it relies upon the laws of supply and demand.

In his landmark essay of 1968[4] Garrett Hardin discusses the tragedy of the commons. Here the commons is a shared grazing area where each cattleman may graze his herd. As each owner expands the herd that grazes upon the commons, the effects of overgrazing become evident and result in a negative impact upon all owners of cattle that graze in this shared space. Yet the cattlemen continue to expand their herds due to the profitability that results from an ever increasing number of cattle. This process continues until the balance between cattle and grazing land is lost, and all suffer. This is Hardin's "tragedy of the commons." So powerful was his original essay that it inspired generations of environmentalists, economists, and biostatisticians who see the world's resources as potential victims of the seemingly unavoidable tragedy that results from the tension between personal gain and resources held in common.

As long as information is viewed merely as a commodity, the economics of supply, demand, and profit will actively work against the idea of open access to information. Logically, the flow of information should not be considered part of the economics of property for the simple reason that, unlike commodities, the production of information is not self-limiting. With the significant exception of paper consumption and reprography, information does not consume in its creation; it creates more information. Information and the knowledge that it creates is a continuing, enriching resource. Unlike the Amazon or Yosemite Valley, it cannot be destroyed by a surplus of visitors or consumers to the information commons. Librarians as a profession have always understood this important aspect of information. They are aware that the more their books are read, the greater the value of the library within the community. Librarians hold as one of their strongest values the concept of access to information for all who need to use it. If access is to be fully realized, it must be linked with the concept of literacy, in both the print and electronic worlds. This concept takes on even greater significance in the digital environment, where access to information may require either professional assistance from a librarian or user training to make the required information accessible.

The areas of government information and the publications resulting from publicly funded research provide the basis for powerful arguments to ensure universal access to this information. Both government information and information derived from research supported by government funding are supported by the public purse. To deny access to these information resources would be to restrict the rights of access to citizens who have, in fact, already paid for this information through their taxes. However, simply opening the doors to these resources is not sufficient. For, in the case of government information, broad-based community access may include documents that are "born digital" as well as the digitization of massive amounts of print information. A computer-literate public with Internet access or technical assistance from a librarian becomes essential. In the case of public access to medical information resulting from research conducted with public funds, the information seeker requires Internet access, some degree of computer literacy, and resources written at a level that is comprehensible. These issues are explored in the chapters on consumer health information and open access. In fact, the idea of promoting information literacy is a necessary condition for access to information in the digital age.

LIBRARIES AND LITERACY

"Universal literacy" like "health for all" resonates as a shining ideal for the improvement of life on this planet. But are these ideals overly ambitious when universal literacy in even the richest countries continues to evade realization? To understand the role of the library and, in particular, the medical library, in working to make these ideals realizable requires an examination of literacy and what literacy means in the information age. We need to revisit the concepts of consumer health, the patient's right to know, and the role of the library in health information literacy.

Literacy resembles second-language acquisition in several important ways. Literacy, like language acquisition, only develops with use—the ability to use a second language improves at an extraordinary rate when the speaker is totally immersed in that language without recourse to the mother tongue. In a second important way, literacy, like second-language acquisition, is a matter of degree. The speaker of a second language may be functionally bilingual—able to buy food and read a letter but not able to discuss sophisticated concepts in the second language. Traditionally, it is educators who have been responsible for developing literacy in the population at large. Libraries have reinforced and encouraged the growth of a reading public, but have not been primarily responsible for teaching reading. However, as information technology became part of the library landscape and as library resources were increasingly provided in the form of digital documents, librarians became involved intensely in instructional programs—known as "information literacy"—in order to make available these new resources. Librarians became intensely engaged in information literacy programs in the 1990s as a necessity since many users lacked the ability to access information without the intervention of the librarian. This practice began gradually, growing out of the traditional instructional programs in bibliography. Librarians had taught users for decades on topics of bibliography, how to access the literature in a particular subject. This was the natural domain of librarians—bibliographic expertise. Originally, card catalogs were a reasonably straightforward tool, requiring little in terms of instruction. However, as card catalogs became the single access point for millions of volumes in large libraries, these too required "decoding." Some of us recall explaining the "divided" (subject versus author-title/catalog) to users and watching their eyes glaze. As for the A.L.A. Filing Rules, carefully imparted to generations of library school students, little need be said!

In the early days of library automation, librarians did their best to make the online catalog resemble in appearance the old catalog card. But as online catalogs were transformed into information systems with powerful links from citation to source documents in the Web environment, research libraries were becoming more sophisticated and also more complex. Even the library's catalog required a level of computer literacy to access library collections. Librarians became increasingly involved in teaching; the title of "instructional services librarian" came into existence, and librarians moved more deeply into their role as educators. The formalization of programs in information literacy has not been without controversy on many university campuses. Perhaps this is the result of the extraordinary zeal with which librarians have responded to this need. Resistance on the part of some faculty may also stem from a desire to maintain control over their domain expertise. The ACRL Guidelines[5] may also appear to some as unduly prescriptive. Finally, the evangelical tone adopted by a few librarians regarding the importance of information literacy programs may not serve the advancement of these programs. These hurdles are challenges to be overcome if librarians are to provide strong programs in information literacy to support access to information.

Literacy and information literacy represent core values in the library profession. But to understand how the values of literacy become operationalized, several distinctions must first be made. All the various "literacies" originate in a firm grounding of reading, be it in the codex or on the computer. The qualification of particular kinds of literacy—subject, cultural, or technical—began to occur gradually, and one of the foremost thinkers to advance a particular form of literacy was E. D. Hirsch.[6] Hirsch writes about the understanding that comes from reading, not about the teaching of reading. Cultural literacy represents the background information that writers assume that readers have. It cannot be achieved by the act of being able to interpret a sequence of letters into a word. In his words:

> Literacy, an essential aim of education in the modern world, is no autonomous empty skill but depends upon literate culture. Like any other aspect of acculturation, literacy requires the early and continued transmission of specific information. Dewey was deeply mistaken to disdain "accumulating information in the form of symbols." Only by accumulating shared symbols, and the shared information that the symbols represent, can we learn to communicate effectively and with one another.[7]

Hirsch well understood the decline of literacy in contemporary culture, and his book remains a *cri de coeur* on behalf of a literate category for improved educational content in school texts.

The publication in 1987 of Hirsch's landmark book is important as well for its temporal context. Ten years earlier, in 1977, *Scientific American* had published its prescient issue devoted to microelectronics.[8] This formidable issue was devoted to explaining to the scientifically literate reader, the development of microelectronics, the art of putting complex electronic circuits on chips of silicon roughly a quarter of an inch square. It presaged the era of the personal computer. The list of contributors to this volume is impressive—including Stan C. Kay, who envisioned that by the 1980s many people would own small computers with the capacity of the large computers available in 1977. In 1983, *Time* magazine was to put a new twist on its "Man of the Year" recognition issue: the computer was *Time's* "Machine of the Year."[9] *Time* made the choice not to designate a single individual, since so many individuals were involved in creating the technological upheaval that was bringing computers to millions. So the "Man of the Year" for 1983 was not a man but the computer itself! During 1982, *Time* had devoted three issues to the revolution that was resulting from computers and had introduced a regular column on computers. Computers were becoming personalized and part of home furnishings. The second major revolution of the 1990s in telecommunications was still ten years in the future, and it is interesting to note how the authors who contributed to this issue were using computer technology, as described in *Time* publisher John A. Myers's words.

> For all that computers have achieved, they can still prove frustrating. In April, Golden's machine inexplicably swallowed the cover story he had written on the Computer Generation. San Francisco correspondent Michael Moritz, part of a special reporting team that included New York Bureau Chief Peter Stoler and Chicago correspondent J. Madelene Nash, briefly lost touch with New York when his telephone computer link malfunctioned. Says contributor Jay Cocks, who anxiously awaited Moritz's report: "They told me that his computer was down. I envisioned an old hippie having a fit of depression. Meanwhile, Senior Writer Otto Friedrich resolutely tapped out his Machine of the Year story on his favourite machine of all—a 15 year old Royal 440.[10]

The benefits of the Internet were still in the future.

Hirsch's cultural literacy did not arise as a reaction to the increasing role of computer technology in all aspects of life. His text does not discuss computers, and he deplores the low level of science teaching in the schools: "So poorly as we have served our students in the humanities and social sciences, we have served them even more poorly in the natural sciences."[11] Hirsch was writing in the decade of the 1980s, a period of sustained growth in knowledge and an increasingly sophisticated technological environment. Although the information society had not yet reached its zenith, the importance of specialized domain knowledge in all fields was growing. Both generalist and specialist were overwhelmed by increasing amounts of information, and to lead an effective life or to practice a profession required literacy, in fact, many different kinds of literacy—cultural, scientific, and numeric. It is in this context that information literacy, one of the dominant "literacies," begins.

HEALTH INFORMATION LITERACY

Health information literacy is part of this general information literacy agenda. It includes aspects of general information literacy programs that are increasingly recognized as core programs and the responsibility of libraries. Health information literacy is itself a broad topic, and in support of the public good it includes service both to students and practitioners in the medical field and to the public at large. Health information literacy includes, first, the education of physicians and their students to access directly scientific information on disease and its treatment. Second, it also includes the development of information for consumers of health care services, such as health promotion information and disease information at a level appropriate to the general public. Third, it includes practical information on health care services in a community or country. Each of these three areas of health information literacy has become a core activity in the work of medical librarians and other practitioners. Through teaching in the classroom and the creation of websites and their validation, medical librarians are providing health information literacy programs as part of formal education programs and a service to their local communities. Health information literacy is examined in detail in part III of this book in the chapters on clinical information and consumer health information.

ENSURING PRESERVATION OF
THE ACCUMULATED WISDOM OF THE PAST

Librarians have taken to heart the Newtonian adage, "If I have seen further it is because I stood on the shoulders of giants." This statement is usually taken at face value, without reflection on the more nuanced interpretation that Newton was in this statement disguising an insult to Robert Hooke, one of his rivals, and a man of short stature. Perhaps Newton was asserting that only selected philosophers (those of a certain stature) had influenced his ideas. Whatever the case, the statement continues to resonate in librarians' thinking as a classic and clear defense of the important influence that writing and thinking from earlier generations continues to have upon the present.

Librarians have taken most seriously their responsibilities for the preservation of the cultural heritage of the past. The digital revolution gave librarians a revitalized and enriched approach to the question of preservation, since in the digital age digital preservation could be linked to access, thus supporting the two core values of providing access to information and preserving the historical record. In the 1990s the mantra of "preservation and access" became a rallying point for the introduction of many of the early digitization projects. Anxious to work with the new technologies, and excited by the possibility of expanding access of scholars to unique materials, these early digitization initiatives brought excitement to the library profession. They served as a source of learning for many librarians, and, more important, they advanced core values. The use of a surrogate copy served to protect fragile original materials from extensive use. As these projects, frequently funded by public grants, proliferated, leadership in setting standards and in the registration of projects and documents became important to avoid duplication of effort and ensure interoperability. Frequently this leadership occurred at the national level, such as the Canadian Initiative on Digital Libraries or the American Memory project of the U.S. Library of Congress, or agencies such as the Council on Library and Information Resources.

Preservation practices in the print world are well developed—appropriate atmospheric conditioning of printed materials; the de-acidification process, including massive de-acidification projects; the use of acid-free materials in the maintenance and binding of collections; and printing on acid-free paper. The campaign of the mid-1980s to convince paper producers and publishers to use acid-free, alkaline paper for publication proved successful. A broad-based awareness program, the "Brittle Book Program," funded by the U.S. National Endowment for the Arts, included the protection of the video "Slow Fires." This campaign had significant impact on the practices of publishers. The U.S. National Library of Medicine, in studying the acid content of the paper publications being added to its collection, reports that only 12 percent of materials continue to carry acidic content, a percentage decline from 80 percent in 1980.[12] These efforts to preserve print-on-paper have been impressive and continue. As the movement becomes a worldwide endeavor, new and improved preservation techniques evolve, and collaboration between libraries grows, such as the joint projects between the National Library of China and the British Library. The task of preserving the cultural heritage in print, including historical medical documents, is enormous, but its dimensions and techniques are understood, and the promise of preserving much of this material exists. The paper codex, if not eternal, is at least a stable medium with fixed text whose physical existence may be assured.

Microfilming of badly deteriorating printed materials is a well-established medium employed by librarians to preserve the intellectual content of endangered, printed materials. In 1986, the U.S. National Library of Medicine began a program of preservation using microfilming of brittle materials to create high-standard microfilm masters to ensure continued access to medical resources. The description on their website serves as a model for intelligent use of microfilm as a preservation strategy:

> Volumes are filmed only if paper breaks at or before two double fields. All volumes are reviewed for artifactual value before filming decisions are made. . . .
>
> NLM's microfilm is produced to the highest technical standards. Stable polyester-based film is used. Volumes that contain important illustrations are filmed in color or continuous tone film to enhance fidelity to the originals. NLM borrows from other libraries' volumes missing from its collections to ensure that filmed runs of serials are as complete as possible. . . . Within copyright restrictions, copies of the film are made available for purchase. . . .
>
> *NLM does not routinely discard volumes prior to filming. Only those volumes judged to be unusable are discarded. This discard rate is less than 10% of all volumes filmed.*[13] (Italics are author's.)

These excerpts provide some degree of assurance regarding the use of microfilming as a preservation strategy for medical literature. North American readers became concerned that libraries may have behaved in a cavalier manner in their approach to their core professional responsibility of preserving the printed records of the past. They were aroused by a highly readable, engaging, and inflammatory book by novelist and *New Yorker* author Nicholson Baker.[14] Baker's book produced a lively, at times almost acrimonious, debate among librarians, historians, and archivists. A number of library educators also engaged in the debate: one of the best summaries of the debate may be found in the Internet journal *First Monday*.[15] Baker condemns the practice of some libraries of microfilming and then discarding the original journal. He too has a commitment to the public good, as evidenced by his bringing these practices to the attention of the public. His would have become a public service, if only Baker had told the story more accurately and less histrionically. A careful reading of Baker's book and the refutation and qualification by Brian Cox's *First Monday* article will, in their totality, do an excellent job of informing the public, at least those interested in the preservation of their cultural heritage, of the complex issues surrounding the preservation of the historical record. Baker has done a fundamental public service in his cautionary tale, which deserves to be required reading of library educators and students in preservation courses, provided Cox's article is also required.

DIGITAL FUTURES FOR PRESERVATION

Digital preservation is an ambiguous concept, for it can refer to the use of digitization technology to preserve and enhance access to material previously in print form. A second meaning to be explored is the necessity of preserving information that exists only in a digital form. Both these definitions are significant for purposes of guaranteeing continuing access to medical information and the culture of health.

Medical libraries have looked historically to technology to enhance and preserve the scholarly record of medicine. There are few medical historical collections today that do not hold copies of facsimile editions of Andreas Vesalius's *De humani corporis fabrica* (1543), reproduced on the four-hundredth anniversary of its first publication, or William Harvey's *De motu cordis* (1628), another four-century-celebrating facsimile. Such fine-quality reproductions were worthy gifts for senior physicians interested in the history of their profession; they also provided the opportunity for libraries and collectors to add these milestone (and costly, rare) items to their collections at a relatively low price; finally, they provided a high-quality, identical copy of the rare volume, thus protecting the original from overuse.

How the world has changed! The scale of access has exploded, enhanced by ever improving scanning technology and the reliability of the Web. A high school student in a small city in the prairies can go online to a website to view the beautiful woodcut illustrations in Vesalius and read the text translated into English.[16] She may also find the magnificent anatomical tables of Bartholomew on the website of the Houston Academy of Medicine McGovern Historical Center[17] for purposes of comparison. These unique historical documents, accompanied by useful, readable commentary, are not, however, an embarrassment of riches. A high school or university student today never knew the pre-Internet world. Not for her the careful scrutiny of bibliographies and the library online catalog! The default for any class assignment is an Internet browser. No need to penetrate the denizens of a library and to seek special permission to consult these valuable sixteenth-century volumes. Although much has been written about the effect of technology on reading, literacy, and the ability to write, these cautionary voices must be at least muted, if not silent, in the face of such extraordinary ease of access to such splendid intellectual resources.

The work of generations of librarians, physicians, and other health professionals reaches fruition in such examples. For centuries, medical libraries and their users have acquired and cherished these documents. Without the generous gift of Harvey Cushing, the historical medical collections of Yale University would be poorer by one hundred fifty volumes in titles published before 1500. And without the extraordinary beneficence of Sir William Osler, McGill's Osler Library of the History of Medicine would, quite simply, not have come into existence. This story of giving and receiving replicates itself in so many other settings, from Newfoundland and the east of North America to the rich historical medical collections at the University of California in Los Angeles and San Francisco. The accumulation of these printed treasures in libraries is now being unlocked in ways that their donors could not have imagined.

What is wrong with this practice? Nothing really, but there are major issues that need to be addressed if this extraordinary benefit made possible by information technology and communications development are to continue to act in the public good. The major issue yet to be solved is that of digital preservation. This problem may best be explored by imagining what the historical medical collections will look like in the year 2050. History of medicine collections have always been built on the foundation of the continuity with medical libraries. Today's science is tomorrow's history, and in fields of accelerated development, that history will be very recent. Various "cutoff" dates are often used to assist in drawing lines of demarcation between past and present: one library may choose the U.S. National Library of Medicine's definition of the literature prior to the beginning of the Great War and use 1913 as the historical point of demarcation; another may choose 1960 as a cutoff date since that is all the material that can be housed in their current site; a third may use the end of each century. Whatever the definition of "historical," all such arbitrary lines are flawed, as any historian knows.

My own prediction is that stewards of medical historical collections will need to consider the advent of electronic medical information as the threshold. This is because this watershed will change the very nature of the historical collection. The designation of runs of journals in print form will no longer await the reader of early issues. Electronic journals began to appear beside their print equivalents in the early 1990s. However, by the turn of the century, most large medical libraries were receiving only electronic versions of these titles. What the historical medical collection will eventually consist of is access to digital versions of *Nature* or *Lancet*. Although the arrival of the digital-only version of medical journals precedes electronic books, many major texts are also being published digitally, especially in the area of multiauthored textbooks and other resources for which currency is a major issue. Documents produced in the creation of new works used to arrive in libraries in boxes with numerous annotations on word-processed printouts, courtesy of the author. Now they are likely to arrive on a compact disc to which the library must provide access. Institutional business, patient records, and government information on health and medical legislation are increasingly in digital forms only.

The public has become accustomed to this in many ways. Indeed, today it is possible to conceptualize an entire medical library as virtual, since almost all the essential clinical information is digital. There is nothing wrong with this picture, provided that the learning curve of the public continues to grow and the teaching of health information literacy remains a priority in the value system of health information professionals. A second proviso is that librarians work to ensure that digital documents are not "here today and gone tomorrow." These are strong requirements, and the faint-hearted best not enter medical librarianship. Although the challenge of digital preservation is a very large one, today's health sciences librarians should take some comfort that there are many strong partners and that much work is already under way, work that will ensure that the medical record will continue to be available. The question of digital preservation is vast, costly, and complex, and many different and powerful allies—major libraries at universities, federal governments, and publishers—are collaborating, experimenting, securing data archives, and sharing their results. The work of the Council on Library and Information Resources is particularly notable for acting as a galvanizing agent in this cause.[18]

The stewardship that underscores the preservation of digital documents will resonate well in many communities, be they librarians, scientists, or the public. There is a growing preference among all constituencies for digital information: it can inform a scientist in the laboratory or at a nursing station in the hospital. It can provide a quick list of nursing homes in a geographic area to an adult whose parents need advice; it can produce a form for tax deduction if a taxpayer is wheelchair bound. While all this information need not be preserved in perpetuity, such examples serve to demonstrate the depth of penetration of health information in digital form in society at large. Those digital resources that require permanent preservation must be carefully selected, and libraries have been choosing materials, and by inference rejecting others, for centuries. In the digital environment, it is possible to consider saving or archiving much more than in the print world. The costs of digital storage decrease at an exponential rate, and the virtual library is unfettered from the limitations of physical volume storage. This possibility, seductive to all collectors, must not detract from the hard work that needs to be done in finding appropriate technological solutions to the need for digital storage and preservation. Real digital preservation requires rigorous and continuing support, in perpetuity, if the public good is to be served. Commitment is essential—as Clifford Lynch stated, "Stewardship is easy and inexpensive to claim; it is expensive and difficult to honor, and perhaps, it will prove to be all too easy to later abdicate."[19]

Health and medical information in support of teaching and research is increasingly digital and relies upon complex and powerful networks. Preservation in this context is profoundly different from the act of preserving print materials, which occurs in individual institutions. The library owns the item to be preserved and takes appropriate steps to guarantee its survival—it is a local decision and the item preserved is owned by the institutions who paid to preserve it. But who pays to preserve a born-digital document that is accessed by the library? Preservation of born-digital documents becomes a consideration at the moment of birth of the document, for there is no waiting period. The digital document will disappear and there will be no fading away, unless one considers unreadable digital documents as "fading." Books, no matter how embrittled, can be read, but digital information requires strategic decisions and alliances as part of the act of creation. It is clear that the exercise of stewardship of medical and health information in the public good is a core value of the practice of medical librarianship. The solutions that are being forged by librarians and other partners are explored in the final chapter of this book.

NOTES

1. Steve Black, "Scholarly Journals Should Be Treated as Public Good," *Serials Librarian* 44, no. 1 (2003): 54.

2. Inge Kaul, ed., *Providing Global Public Goods: Managing Globalization*, published for the United Nations Development Programme (New York: Oxford University Press, 2003), 44.

3. Michael Gorman, *Our Enduring Values: Librarianship in the 21st Century* (Chicago: American Library Association, 2000).

4. Garrett Hardin, "The Tragedy of the Commons," *Science* 162 (1968): 1243–48.

5. *Information Literacy Competency Standards for Higher Education* (Chicago: American Library Association, 2000).

6. E. D. Hirsch, *Cultural Literacy: What Every American Needs to Know* (Boston: Houghton Mifflin, 1987).

7. Hirsch, *Cultural Literacy*, xvii.

8. *Scientific American*, 237, no. 1 (September 1977).

9. Otto Friedrich, "Machine of the Year: The Computer Moves In," *Time* (January 3, 1983).

10. *Time*, "Machine of the Year," iii.

11. Hirsch, *Cultural Literacy*, 147.

12. U.S. National Library of Medicine, Preservation Policy, http://www.nlm.nih.gov.psd/pcm/nlmpres.htm (accessed September 20, 2004).

13. U.S. National Library of Medicine, Preservation Practices, http://www.nlm.nih.gov.psd/pcm/nlmprespract.html (accessed September 20, 2004).

14. Nicholson Baker, *Double Fold: Libraries and the Assault on Paper* (New York: Random House, 2001).

15. Richard J. Cox, "The Great Newspaper Caper; Backlash in the Digital Age," *First Monday*, http://firstmonday.org.issues/issues 5-12/cox/index/html (accessed September 23, 2004). Cox has developed these ideas in his book *Vandals in the Stacks: A Response to Baker's Assault on Libraries* (Westport, CT: Greenwood, 2002).

16. Northwestern University, http://vesalius.northwestern.edu/index.html (accessed September 24, 2004).

17. Houston Academy of Medicine, Texas Medical Center Library, http://mcgovern.library.tmc.edu/anatomy/eustachi/contents-htm/ (accessed September 24, 2004).

18. Council on Library and Information Resources, "Access in the Future Tense," http://www.clir.org (accessed September 30, 2004).

19. Clifford A. Lynch, "Institutional Repositories: Essential Infrastructure for Scholarship in the Digital Age," *ARL Bimonthly Report* 226, http://www.ar.org.newsltr/236/ir.html.

II

THE ORIGIN OF MEDICAL LIBRARIANSHIP

2

EARLY DAYS IN THE PROFESSION

This chapter considers the development of medical librarianship within a relatively recent and essentially North American context. Medical librarianship developed within the culture of medicine, and the demands created by improvements in the teaching and practice of medicine resulted in enhanced roles for the medical library. Developments in international medical librarianship are considered within the context of the International Congresses on Medical Librarianship.

THE DEVELOPMENT OF THE MEDICAL PROFESSION:
ITS IMPACT ON MEDICAL LIBRARIES

Medicine, arguably the oldest of the professions, has a well-documented history recorded in the extensive historical collections throughout the developed world. Collections such as those housed at the U.S. National Library of Medicine, the Countway Library's History of Medicine Division at Harvard University, the Wellcome Institute for the History of Medicine in London, and the Osler Library of the History of Medicine at McGill University in Montreal, to name only a few, document the development of medical progress over millennia. These collections are frequently supported and cherished by members of the medical profession who, especially in their senior years, display keen and sustained interest in their profession.

The certification and licensing of medical practitioners does not manifest the same coherence as the development of the discipline of medicine. Lacking an internal scientific logic and strongly impacted by social forces, the certification of practitioners of medicine in North America demonstrates the characteristics of a profession that is constantly evolving in response to social forces and an ever increasing knowledge base. The development of medical librarianship evolved from the same social, political, legal, and economic crucible that gave rise to North American medical practice. Specialization in medical librarianship evolved, much as did specialization in medicine in the nineteenth century, as a specialization within the field. Medical librarianship was responding to a growing need to provide specialized library service to the medical profession, which was itself evolving and laying claim to a position of eminence in the hierarchy of the professions.

The American sociologist Paul Starr has described the social origins of American medical practice, and he identifies the conditions that were essential to the development of the medical profession. Starr emphasizes a profession's ability to lay claim to professional authority as essential to its success; by claiming authority and having that authority respected, a dependence upon the profession is created in the society at large. The claim to authority certainly serves as a necessary condition for all professions, indeed for trades as well as professions. A plumber or a systems administrator may also lay claim to authority. We are all aware of the authority demonstrated by those who work in these fields. But professional authority involves further claims, according to Starr: "First, the knowledge and competence of the profession have been validated by the community of his or her peers; second, that this consensually validated knowledge and competence rest on rational, scientific grounds; and third, that the professional's judgment and advice are oriented toward a set of values, such as health."[1] These three criteria of knowledge, validation, and values are the origin of the collegial, cognitive, and moral characteristics of a mature profession. Starr develops these themes in his analysis of the growth and establishment of the medical profession, showing how they ensured the professional sovereignty that medicine attained throughout North America.

Evolving from small, private medical colleges in antebellum America, medical education and practice arrived at its preeminent position in American society through a continuing upgrading of the profession. These improvements were sustained and comprehensive: in education by prolonging the training period for entry into the profession, in developing identity and collegiality among students, in controlling the quality and quantity of individuals certified for practice, and by developing powerful agencies such as the American Medical Association and its Council on Medical Education to ensure quality and control within the profession of medicine. Starr shows that, as the authority of the medical profession expanded, the need for more resources to support the profession, both in education and practice, grew.

This is particularly interesting, as it helps to explain the growth and improvement in academic medical libraries as well as the rise of medical librarianship. As medicine became more professionalized and medical training more rigorous, the role of the medical library in providing access to established knowledge became recognized. In particular, the evolution of the U.S. National Library of Medicine demonstrates the recognition of the importance of access to medical information.

Is it possible to evaluate medical librarianship according to the collegial, cognitive, and value-driven criteria identified by Starr as essential to the establishment of medical authority? Collegiality, authority, and the validation of knowledge and competence by a community of peers form the basis of the professional education of librarians and their socialization into the profession. Entry into the profession of librarianship normally requires a graduate degree from a school of library or information studies associated with a university. These programs of study are currently reviewed and evaluated at regular intervals by the Committee on Accreditation of the American Library Association. In the process, library practitioners and educators, established and recognized in their field, are invited to participate in intensive reviews of library and information studies programs at the university. A review team evaluates the program according to goals identified by the school being reviewed and established criteria such as course content, research, teaching, and support services. Accreditation is given or withheld based upon the visiting team's evaluation of the program. Collegial authority is deeply embedded in this reviewing process. This accreditation process is concerned, however, with education for librarianship in general; it is not an evaluation of medical librarianship. In fact, no clear path exists in library education for the development of competency in medical librarianship. A number of graduate programs in library education may offer a course or two in medical librarianship, or more recently in medical information resources, medical informatics, or evidence-based medicine. But these course offerings are frequently on an ad hoc basis, dependent upon the willingness of a local practicing medical librarian to teach the course, and there are no prerequisites for enrollment in these courses. The conclusion is clear: while there is collegial authority in the review of education for librarianship in general, formal education for medical librarianship is not well developed and does not demonstrate continuing review by peers.

To correct this deficit in the field, the Medical Library Association (Chicago), the Canadian Health Libraries Association, and other associations of medical librarians outside North America offer numerous workshops and training sessions. These courses are well attended by medical librarians.

Instructors are evaluated, but usually there is no evaluation of learning outcomes on the part of participants. Another form of collegial review has been implemented by the Medical Library Association. Through its Academy of Health Information Professionals, it reviews the education and professional contribution of self-selected applicants for the academy, ranking them according to preestablished criteria. Membership in the academy is viewed as desirable, but has not succeeded as an essential criterion for medical library practice.

The second criterion, cognitive authority, requires the acquisition of a body of knowledge and competence based upon rational, scientific method. This criterion raises the lingering question of whether librarianship is in fact a science and whether there exists a body of cognitive knowledge on which the field rests. Certainly, medical librarianship consists of a well-codified set of increasingly sophisticated practices that constitute good medical librarianship. The Medical Library Association has done sustained and groundbreaking work over decades in publishing its *Handbooks*, which provide a summary of state-of-the-art best practices. Research in the field is well documented and peer reviewed in a number of publications, but chiefly the *Journal of the Medical Library Association*. However, cognitive authority requires a firm foundation of education before the professional education of the practitioner begins. Clearly this cannot take place in a discipline for which the formal education is at best limited to a few ad hoc courses. The required education for librarianship in general is a nonthesis master's degree, which in the majority of North American schools is completed within a twelve-month period. Despite the devotion to continuing education and dedicated service, medical librarians are not provided with a strong cognitive base for entering the profession. The fact that this professional specialty has emerged into a successful and attractive career path may be attributed to the men and women who have provided strong role models and inspired on-the-job learning. The need for greater domain knowledge in education for medical librarianship may also account for new professionals entering the field of medical librarianship. As medical libraries entered the information age, medical informatics emerged, providing educational opportunities that merged medical science, information technology, and information science. The medical informationist, a concept that is explored in detail later in this volume, is part of the current medical library environment. Medical informatics is another specialization and one that is built upon a strong foundation of medical training; medical informatics specialists are beginning to hold positions at the level of associate dean in faculties of medicine and frequently have responsibility for the academic medical library.

Starr's final criterion, professional authority, rests upon the professional practitioner's judgment and is an expression of clearly articulated values. On this third criterion, medical librarianship may lay its strongest claim. We have identified in the preceding chapter the core values of the profession—access to health information, health information literacy, and the guarantee of secure and available access to the literature of the biomedical sciences. These core values share a common characteristic: they derive their meaning from actions that implement those values. They express the belief that certain things must be done, and a commitment that certain problems must be investigated. There is an imperative about both action and investigation, and in the case of the core values of medical librarianship, the emphasis is upon the action. Medical librarianship is the implementation of practices that support these core values. The result of these practices is a profession that has fully internalized these core values, and in so doing, acts "in the public good."

By the end of the twentieth century, medicine had emerged as the paradigmatic profession in North America. The challenge of acceptance into medicine and the rigor of the educational programs have resulted in eminent social and economic status for the successful medical graduate. No other profession has been able to achieve this recognition. But medical librarianship, a distinct profession but practiced within the medical profession, does not enjoy the same authority or economic rewards that characterize the medical profession. Neither do other valuable professions such as physical therapy or nursing. However, through the intellectual and cultural iconography of the library, medical librarians have occupied a unique and relatively privileged role. The authority of the library rests upon its guardianship of the intellectual history of medicine combined with the provision of access to the most recent information on advances in medical science. The authority of the library still has the power to create respect in the first-year student, whose education begins and continues in the library, be it print or digital.

THE ESTABLISHMENT OF
LIBRARIANSHIP IN NORTH AMERICA

In the nineteenth century, the number of institutions of higher education in Canada and the United States was growing. As universities expanded, teachers and students required increasingly large library collections. These collections were frequently under the charge of a scholar without library training. Yet with the exception of an apprenticeship at a well-established library, there existed no educational opportunities for learning to be a librarian. When the American Civil War ended, the United States witnessed unparalleled social and economic expansion, giving rise not only to further expansion of universities and their libraries, but to the availability of libraries for the general public.

The philanthropy of Andrew Carnegie is one of the single strongest determinants of the growth of public libraries. During his lifetime, Carnegie endowed some twenty-five hundred libraries throughout the English-speaking world in the United States, Canada, Australia, New Zealand, South Africa, the West Indies, and Europe. Within Canada, the first Carnegie library was the Vancouver Public Library, which opened to the public in 1903. Among numerous Carnegie grant libraries in Canada is the original library building for the Ottawa Public Library in Canada's national capital. In Carnegie grant libraries, the municipality took responsibility for the library site and maintenance once a library was built, since Carnegie did not provide for continuing funding. Carnegie's "rags to riches" life and his commitment to pay back to society his good fortune is a familiar story told on a grand scale. What is less well known is the fact that Andrew Carnegie, in addition to giving to library development, was also the single biggest donor to the New York Society for the Suppression of Vice.[2] Libraries would provide reading materials that were morally upright, an effective and available alternative to the salacious materials that led to anti-obscenity legislation in the English-speaking world. In the United States, the Comstock Act of 1865 was aimed especially at the transportation of obscene books (including information on birth control and abortion), but by inference it would shape the nature and development of collections in public libraries for many years. In a sense, the establishment of public libraries had a moral imperative, not only in the sense of Horatio Alger, but also as a means of enforcing through the collections certain moral standards. The library was part of the community support to maintain the moral character of its citizens. If, as argued in chapter one, one of the core values of the professional librarian is the provision of access to information and the affirmation of the rights of users without censorship, the ambivalence between "moral" collections and the rights of the citizen to access information placed the librarian in a difficult position.

The growth of both public and university libraries in the nineteenth century created the necessary conditions for the establishment of an association that would provide a forum for the sharing of knowledge among members of the incipient profession. The American Library Association came into existence in 1876; the Library Association (Great Britain) in 1877. The Canadian Library Association, by contrast, was established much later, in 1946, probably a reflection of the strong contribution and involvement of Canadian librarians in American associations. The centennial year of the United States of America has been described as the year that librarianship laid claim to being a profession.[3]

JOHN SHAW BILLINGS AND THE *INDEX-CATALOGUE* OF THE SURGEON GENERAL'S OFFICE

The practice of librarianship rests on a strong commitment to bibliography. In medical librarianship, the development of medical bibliography has deep historical roots, originating in the early days of printing. In her foundation study of medical bibliography,[4] Estelle Brodman distinguishes between the early centuries, from the sixteenth to the mid-nineteenth century, described as the age of individual medical bibliographers and the growth of cooperative bibliography, especially the creation of Royal Society of London's *Catalogue*, and the *Index-Catalogue* of the Office of the Surgeon General. This latter effort, despite the fact that it was a cooperative effort, is closely linked with one unusual individual, John Shaw Billings.

If "public good" is served by providing access to health care, it follows that health and healing are advanced by access to the medical literature. In nineteenth-century America, this connection was strongly established through the work of John Shaw Billings and the creation of a national medical library. Through incremental growth and the determination of Billings, what began as a few books in the doctor's office became today's world leader in access to the literature of biomedicine.

The American Civil War created demands for the most current medical information by medical officers in the fields of surgery, medication, and clinical therapy, and required access to a growing number of medical journals published in the United States and Europe. It is difficult to imagine what was meant by access to medical information in this era, in large measure because of the quality, convenience, and reliability of medical information that exists today. During the Civil War access to medical information meant the purchase of multiple copies of medical books by the library and their distribution to physicians working in the field. Among the titles purchased in duplicate by the Surgeon General's Office during the Civil War were Bumstead's *Venereal Disease* (7,317 copies), Eriksen's *Surgery* (5,370 copies), the *Dispensatory of the United*

States (4,850 copies), Gray's *Anatomy* (3,442 copies) and Dunglison's *Medical Dictionary* (1,905 copies).[5]

The Library of the Surgeon General's Office continued to expand, and, to the good fortune of medical librarianship, saw the arrival of assistant army surgeon John Shaw Billings in 1864.[6] He was to serve the library from 1865 to 1895. Billings's first assignment in the office was the management of civilian physicians engaged in the war effort, and, subsequently, the phasing out of military hospitals once the war ended. But growing needs in Washington required administrative attention, and Billings was shortly appointed as the officer in charge of the Library of the Surgeon General's Office. He was to hold this responsibility during a period of unprecedented growth and development in medicine and in the American economy. Among his many significant achievements was the idea of outreach by the library to the physician in the field. Under Billings, the library expanded its mandate to include physicians in general, not only the military. He addressed the need to access the current medical literature by publicizing the existence of the library and the broad distribution of the library's book catalog. During the years following the Civil War, the library was launched as a public institution, providing relevant information to the medical profession.

Billings demonstrated extraordinary diligence in acquiring materials for his collection. He shared all the compulsion of a true collector in building the collection and in using volunteers, mainly physicians, to track down important "desiderata" items. He was particularly diligent in tracking back issues of medical journals to ensure that the library retained a complete run of a periodical title. And his efforts were not limited to American titles. Billings was concerned to acquire the first Canadian medical periodical *Journal de médecine de Québec* (1826–1827). George E. Fenwick, professor of surgery at the Montreal General Hospital, was contacted, as was John Fulton, professor of physiology at Trinity College Medical School in Toronto and editor of *Canada Lancet*. Editors of medical and dental journals were on Billings's "hit list" and he achieved considerable success in his work with Canadian medical authors, editors, and practitioners as well as with physicians in the United States.

Editors seem to have been particularly helpful in Canada, where Billings had no medical officers serving as part-time book scouts. John Fulton published Billings's letter in *Canada Lancet* and thereby brought donations and exchanges from cooperative Canadians—J. E. Fitzpatrick from Baie-St-Paul, Quebec, sent rare Quebec journals, annuaires of Laval University, and other publications. H. J. Saunders, Kingston, Ontario, sent volume 6 of *Medical Chronicle or Montreal Monthly Journal of Medical and Physical Science* in exchange for circulars of the Surgeon General's Office.[7] Billings's success outside the United States had important implications for access to medical literature worldwide and anticipates the role that library was to play in serving the public good through acquiring and providing access to medical information on an international scale.

John Shaw Billings was the right man, in the right place at the right time. He grasped the importance of acquiring a comprehensive collection of medical information at a time when the literature of medicine was expanding both in North America and Europe. He understood the importance of a central, federally funded agency to ensure that the literature was used in the service of the public good. And, perhaps most significantly for the future program of the U.S. National Library of Medicine, he was determined to provide comprehensive, detailed, bibliographic control of the literature that he was acquiring with singled-minded determination. Billings had already provided the library with a book catalog organized by authors, but the important problem of accessing the medical literature in journal form had yet to be tackled. Both Brodman and Miles have identified the appearance of the *Catalogue of Scientific Papers* of the Royal Society of London in 1867 as an important first step in bringing the scientific journal literature under control. Billings wanted a subject index as well as an author approach to the literature, recognizing the importance the subject approach in clinical medicine would have, and in 1874 he set out to provide this access.

His creative and productive approach to the development of the first volume of the *Index-Catalogue* of the Surgeon General's Library has been fully described by Estelle Brodman. In the creation of his bibliography, Billings did not have at his disposal professional medical librarians to assist in the monumental task that lay ahead of him. Even if a well-trained cadre of medical librarians had existed at the time, it is doubtful that Billings would have availed himself of this opportunity. His approach was to be both highly personal and professional. The cooperative aspect of the bibliography rested in his use of a team of clerical assistants, including the volunteer efforts of wives of staff, and, as the burden of subject analysis grew, the enlistment of physicians to assist in the work of subject analysis. He insisted on exercising quality control personally as he reviewed all current journals received in his library, indicating which ones should be included in the *Index-Catalogue* and, according to Garrison, established high criteria for inclusion, failing, in one instance, to include a case study of acute rheumatism by William Jenner and a compound fracture treated by the Lister method.[8]

Billings's work was lessened somewhat with the arrival of a trusted assistant, Robert Fletcher, who served as his assistant librarian. Billings created an economy of labor that recycled the indexing for the *Index-Catalogue* into the production of the *Index Medicus*. He also delegated some of the work on the *Index Medicus* to Fletcher, who approached his task in a more comprehensive and less critical manner. The result was that the *Index Medicus* approached comprehensive coverage, and the *Index-Catalogue* was more selective and quality controlled. The issue of quality control continued as an important consideration in the production of the *Index Medicus* into the computer age, with the careful and critical selection of journals for inclusion. Today, the inclusion of a journal in the *Index Medicus* virtually guarantees that it will be perceived as a significant title, and included in journals packaged for electronic publishing.

Before the monumental task of subject analysis began, there had been earlier author listings of volumes in the Library of the Surgeon General's Office. The first catalog for which Billings was himself responsible appeared in 1873[9] and recorded twenty-five thousand volumes and fifteen thousand pamphlets, but this record did not provide the necessary detailed subject analysis of the journal literature that Billings was convinced was essential:

> In a majority of cases what [the physicians] want are the statistics of a given disease, operation or remedy. The data for these statistics are for the most part contained in journals and transactions of societies. To make these available, a card catalogue of all important papers in such journals and transactions has been prepared.[10]

Before he could begin his task, Billings had to obtain the necessary government funding, and to convince the Appropriations Committee of the U.S. Congress of the need to allocate funds for this purpose. Billings prepared a sample of the proposed catalog, a *Specimen Fasciculus*, which was initially distributed to physicians and librarians for their comments, and, of course, their support in the intensive effort to raise funds for this initiative. Billings's efforts were rewarded in 1879 when Congress approved funding for his work, and in 1880 the first volume (A–Belinski) appeared, with subsequent volumes appearing until the alphabet was completed in 1895 when Billings retired from the army. Fletcher continued to follow the pattern of publication established by Billings, but it was becoming evident that the *Index-Catalogue* could not be sustained perpetually, and the monumental series eventually came to closure. It was left to the *Index Medicus* and its successive iterations to continue the comprehensive and reliable coverage of the medical literature that Billings had begun. The tremendous burgeoning of the medical literature of the late nineteenth and twentieth century and the costs of production of the catalog had brought this distinguished sequence of catalogs to a halt. But not before several efforts were made for continuation, including a fourth series that was discontinued with volume ten. The *Index Medicus* continued to be present as an effective tool for accessing the medical literature throughout the world.

Billings had tamed the tiger of comprehensive medical bibliography and in the process changed fundamentally the work of medical librarians. He wrote the agenda for the future transformation of the Library of the Surgeon General's Office to today's U.S. National Library of Medicine—to acquire and make available reliable medical information to the medical profession. His contribution is all the more significant in the context of the other major roles he undertook as director of the New York Public Library (1896–1913) and president of the American Library Association (1901–1902).

THE BIRTH OF THE MEDICAL LIBRARY ASSOCIATION

The nineteenth century witnessed the increasing professionalization of medical education and the practice of medicine. Following the end of the American Civil War, access to medical information advanced largely through the leadership of the Surgeon General's Office and the development of its *Index-Catalogue*. A final major development was essential: the formalization of the practice of medical librarianship and its advancement through the founding in 1898 of the Medical Library Association. Three strong-minded professionals, one librarian and two physicians, brought the association into existence: Sir William Osler (1849–1919), George Milbry Gould (1848–1922), and Margaret Charlton (1850–1931).

Osler began his medical studies at Toronto Medical School, but later switched to McGill University because of the superior clinical opportunities it offered. He graduated from McGill in 1872, studied in Europe for several years, and returned to accept an appointment at McGill as lecturer in the Institutes of Medicine. While a lecturer at McGill, Osler traveled to the United States, in particular in 1876 to Boston to use the Boston Medical Library for material on clinical subjects not available at McGill. In 1881, on behalf of McGill University, Osler attended the International Medical Congress in London, where it is likely that he met John Shaw Billings. Following this meeting, Osler was in touch with Billings, providing material for the Library of the Surgeon General's Office.

In 1884, Osler left Montreal to accept the chair of clinical medicine at the University of Pennsylvania. Before he left Montreal, he gave his journal collection to the McGill Medical Library. In Philadelphia, Osler became a member of the College of Physicians of Philadelphia, and had access to its great library. Osler was a familiar figure in this library, serving on its Library Committee, and was well known as a prowler of the stacks:

> He . . . habitually prowled amongst its treasures . . . instead of keeping office hours or seeing private patients. An "important engagement" often was kept with old favourites on the library shelves. So well did he get to know the library's contents that he was able to write from Baltimore several years later as to just where to find some duplicate odd volumes of the *Transactions of the Philadelphia Pathological Society* that he wanted for the Library of the Medical and Chirurgical Faculty.[11]

Four years after his arrival in Philadelphia, Osler was invited to become chief of staff at the Johns Hopkins University and Hospital in Baltimore. It is probable that the friendship begun with Billings in London while Osler was still at McGill had influenced this outcome: Billings was medical adviser to the Johns Hopkins Hospital Board. Billings had visited Osler at his rooms in Philadelphia on Walnut Street to consult with him regarding the appointment at Johns Hopkins, and in May 1889, Osler assumed his new duties in Baltimore. Billings and Osler were united again as Osler now had easy access to the Surgeon General's Library in Washington. On one occasion, Billings reminded Osler of his tardiness in returning a book and William Osler replied, "Bring a club with you in your next visit and pummel me, well. Yes do order the book and make me pay double for it, if possible. What an aggravating devil I am!"[12]

Predictably, in Baltimore, Osler's interests and zeal fell upon the then moribund Library of the Medical and Chirurgical Faculty of the State of Maryland, housed in the basement at the Maryland Historical Society. He became a member of its library committee on which he served until he left for England in 1905. He saw the library grow from a few hundred volumes to some fifteen thousand by 1905. More importantly for the history of the association, in 1896 he was influential in the appointment of the library's first professional librarian, Marcia C. Noyes, who continued to be associated with it until her death in 1946.

Osler's career culminated in his appointment as Regius Professor of Medicine at Oxford in 1905, a post previously held by John Burdon Sanderson, who had taught Osler thirty-four years earlier. Happily for

Osler, his responsibilities included a curatorship in the Bodleian Library. Here Osler continued his strong support of libraries by acquiring material and by donating to the library. At Oxford, Osler's vision and sense of importance of books and libraries reached new heights. Although he did not realize this goal, Osler, according to Cushing, envisioned

> a college where men could learn everything relating to the Book, from the preparation of manuscript and the whole mystery of authorship to the art of binding; everything from the manufacturing of paper to the type with which the book is printed; everything related to the press and to the mart; everything about the history of printing from Gutenberg . . . how to stack and store books; how to catalogue, how to distribute them; how to make them vital living units in a community. There should be such a College and it should be at Oxford.[13]

Osler's contribution as a teacher and educator united with his love of learning—his passion to know and his willingness to share his knowledge. He knew the importance of quiet study and, in one of his most memorable sayings, commented that "to study the phenomena of disease without books is to sail an uncharted sea, while to study books without patients is not to go to sea at all." In 1892, Osler presented the medical world with the first edition of his *The Principals and Practice of Medicine* to claim a strong position for North American medicine, through its heavy reliance on Canadian and American authors. This work was a unique contribution to the field of medical texts and was renowned for its systematization of diseases. It became a standard reference source for librarians and bibliographers, with its outstanding chapters on the fields of contagion and diseases of the heart and circulatory system, as well as its numerous classical and literary allusions. Osler's text was published in sixteen editions over a period of fifty-five years. It remains as a living reminder of Osler's scholarly breadth and the depth of his learning.[14] Osler's commitment to medical libraries was lifelong and the effect he had on librarians is captured in these reminiscences of Minnie Wright Blogg, who knew Osler when she was librarian at Johns Hopkins Hospital during Osler's tenure in Baltimore.

> The present Librarian of the Johns Hopkins Hospital, entering upon her duties twenty years ago . . . found herself overwhelmed with work, and one day, arranging books and journals came to a point where she settled herself comfortably on the floor . . . she was alone in the Library, and was absorbed in arranging the hundreds of journals and reprints which surrounded her. Suddenly, she became aware of a light,

rapid step approaching and almost immediately there appeared in the doorway a man who paused and looked at her. Distinguished, keen, slight and wonderfully alert, he stood; he wore a black frock coat, carried a silk hat and gaily swung a slender cane. We looked at each other; neither spoke. Then in a singularly kind and sympathetic voice . . . he asked, "Is this the new Librarian?" I could not deny it.[15]

Few physicians have made a more important impact upon the development of medical libraries than did Sir William Osler.

Scores there are, and have been, that have left an imprint upon one medical library, and there are some whose influence has extended to two or three, but Sir William Osler is the only one whose magic has touched all. Wherever he happened to be, his interest in the medical library was paramount.[16]

During his life Osler gave generously to a number of libraries, including, but not limited to, those of the institutions with whom he was associated. Libraries benefiting from his generosity included the Library of the Surgeon General's Office, the Bodleian Library, the Library of the College of Physicians, the Library of the Medical and Chirurgical Faculty of the University of Maryland, the Library of Johns Hopkins Hospital, the Academy of Medicine of Toronto and, foremost among this group, McGill University, his alma mater. Osler understood that a good library had to be financially healthy; he gave generously and encouraged others to do the same.

His most enduring gift, that of his personal library, to the Faculty of Medicine of McGill University, speaks to his thoughtfulness as much as to his generosity. In his own words, he shows himself an early advocate of resource sharing: "I should like to have been able to leave my collection to the [Johns Hopkins] School, but it seems more appropriate to give it to McGill where it is much more needed. After all, for the older and rarer books the Hopkins has the Surgeon General's Library at its door."[17]

Despite his decision to donate to McGill, Osler continued his interest in other libraries. Just one year before his death, he wrote to Margaret Charlton, at the Academy of Medicine in Toronto:

I hope your library grows. I have some duplicates to send you when opportunity offers. . . . Are you trying to collect all details about the local profession? . . . You should start a special section of the library if you have not already done so, dealing with Ontario medical history— pictures, books, pamphlets, letters, diplomas, etc. I enclose you $100 to be spent by the Library Committee in this work.[18]

As a collector and donor, Osler was both generous and slightly forget-ful. In 1907, he presented McGill with a 1543 Vesalius only to have the li-brarian point out an even better copy on display, which Osler had given to the library some years earlier. Osler determined then that he would give the copy to the Boston Medical Library. On presenting the volume, the Boston librarian showed Osler yet another 1543 Vesalius, which Osler had previ-ously presented to that library. The Vesalius finally found a home in the Li-brary of the New York Academy of Medicine.

Bibliographic access and physical access were matters of great concern to Osler. Reading current medical literature was for Osler essential to pa-tient care. As he put it,

> It is hard for me to speak of the value of libraries in terms which would not seem exaggerated. . . . For the teacher and the worker a great li-brary . . . is indispensable. They must know the world's best work and know it at once. They mint and make current coin the ore so widely scattered in journals, transactions and monographs.[19]

This emphasis on the need to know, to have access to the best and to have it immediately, is a recurring theme in the work of Osler. It is evident in his emphasis on the importance of knowing the current medical litera-ture through the various journal clubs that he established at the institutions where he held positions. In his words, "It is in utilizing the fresh knowledge of the journals that the young physician may attain quickly to the name and fame he desires."[20] Osler wrote with dramatic effect of the problems cre-ated for the library and the user by the rapid obsolescence of medical in-formation:

> It is sad to think how useless are a majority of the works on our shelves—the old cyclopedias and dictionaries, the files of defunct jour-nals, the endless editions of text-books as dead as their authors. Only a few epoch-making works survive. . . . Now among the colossal mass of rubbish on the shelves there are some precious gems which should be polished and well set and in every library put out on view.[21]

Osler is the most renowned of the association's three founders. Un-fortunately, the last years of his life at Oxford were marked by sadness. Later in life he married a widow, Grace Revere Gross, and their one son, Revere, was killed in World War I. Throughout all of life's experiences, Osler continued to renew himself through reading. In his career, his teaching, his writing, and his medical consulting, he placed enormous emphasis on books and libraries. That he became one of the three founding members of the Medical Library Association is a predictable consequence of this emphasis.

George Milbry Gould, along with William Osler, was responsible for the creation of the Medical Library Association. Gould was described in an obituary as "a man of lofty principles, wide and varied learning, a white hot zeal, unflagging energy, and a warm and constant heart."[22] After a childhood spent in Athens, Ohio, he became a drummer boy in the Civil War, serving in the Sixty-third Regiment of the Ohio Volunteers from 1861 to 1862 and later as a volunteer in the One Hundred Forty-first Ohio Volunteers Infantry. Perhaps it was the war experience that led him to study briefly at Harvard Divinity School and ultimately, following a time as owner of a bookstore, to study medicine at Jefferson Medical College. He graduated in 1889—by that time he was forty years old—and immediately opened an ophthalmology office in Philadelphia at 119 South Seventeenth Street, with a private residence at 1722 Walnut Street in the city. Gould's interest in books and publishing converged on the literature of medicine, and he edited the *Medical News*, 1891–1895; the *Philadelphia Medical Journal*, 1898–1900; and *American Medicine*, 1901–1906. During his career, numerous offices and honors were offered him. He wrote extensively in his medical speciality of ophthalmology, but he is best remembered as a medical lexicographer through his *Students' Medical Dictionary*, *Practitioner's Medical Dictionary*, and *Pocket Medical Dictionary*. His medical dictionaries sold more than one half million copies, and he was also a prolific author of literary works, including a book of poems (1897) and a biography of Lafcadio Hearn (1908).

As an ophthalmologist, he is remembered for his career in detecting errors of refraction to aid in relieving eye strain, from which he himself suffered. In his "Biographic Clinics" he concludes that the poor health of many famous people was due to eye strain. Gould had a broad intellectual curiosity, writing on such questions as why sap rises in trees, the reasons for the shape of shells, and library questions. His writings and the variety of his intellectual interests made him strongly reliant upon libraries throughout his professional career. It was predictable that, like Osler, he would have recognized and actively supported the founding of an association of medical librarians.

The final member of the founding triumvirate, Margaret Ridley Charlton, medical librarian and medical historian, is the least well known. In 1895, in her thirty-seventh year, Margaret Charlton was engaged by the Faculty of Medicine of McGill University to work in the faculty library.

When she came to the library, it was already seventy-two years old and the largest in North America connected with a medical school. At the time, it contained fourteen thousand volumes, and during her nineteen-year tenure, ten thousand volumes were added. Margaret Charlton entered the profession of librarianship following a career in literary journalism in which she wrote numerous historical sketches for the *Dominion Illustrated Monthly* and several books.[23] In entering librarianship she was ahead of her time, for at the end of the last century librarianship as a profession for women had not developed to any extent. By the standards of genteel ladies of her day, she was well educated for the position, having attended the Montreal High School and a summer course in librarianship at Amherst College in Amherst, Massachusetts, where Melvil Dewey taught. In his presidential address to the Medical Library Association in 1936, W. W. Francis, the first Osler Librarian, described her as "thoroughly imbued, perhaps . . . be-Dewied with his classification."[24]

Charlton remained as assistant medical librarian at McGill until 1914, when she resigned to take charge of the Academy of Medicine Library in Toronto. We do not know the precise conditions of her initial appointment at McGill in 1895. By 1896, however, she was already interested in library work beyond her immediate place of employment, for the Minutes of the Library Committee of the Faculty of Medicine[25] record a reimbursement of fifty-five dollars for her expenses in attending a meeting of the American Library Association in Chicago. For nineteen years Charlton was assistant medical librarian to the honorary medical librarian, Frederick Gault Finley, who held this post from 1895 until 1914. As practicing assistant medical librarian, Charlton must have enjoyed the support and encouragement of Finley, whose term as honorary librarian overlapped so closely with her own period at McGill.

All was not harmony within the library, however; William Francis, Osler Librarian, noted in his 1936 Presidential Address to the Medical Library Association that "a sensitive, book-devouring investigator was disliked by and positively afraid of our mild librarian! For though there was always a quiet dignity about Miss Charlton, it did not conceal her fervid likes and dislikes."[26] There was, however, more at stake than the personal preferences of Miss Charlton. In 1908, the Minutes of the Library Committee of the Faculty of Medicine of McGill University stated, "The Assistant Librarian's attention should be drawn to the laxity with which journals are taken out by members of the staff and not recorded. . . . That, moreover, it is essential that civility be shown to all who decide to make use of the Library."[27] By 1912 the dissatisfaction with Charlton's management appears to have reached a peak. The Library Committee Minutes again express the concerns as follows: "The cataloguing was very far behind and . . . was not keeping pace with the accessions. As to the bookkeeping, there were serious complaints that this was badly muddled. There was more than a suspicion that accounts had been not infrequently twice paid."[28]

By this time, the staff of the library, in addition to Charlton, consisted of two full-time assistants and a third half-time assistant. The committee recommended that the two full-time assistants be dismissed and replaced by a second assistant librarian, equal in status to Charlton, who would be in charge of correspondence, the lending library, and the reading room. By the end of 1914, Charlton had left the McGill Medical Library. Years later, in 1936, Finley, who had been honorary librarian, wrote in a letter to Francis: "I held on to the post of Hon. Librarian long after I should have resigned as I knew that few others would have tolerated her [Charlton's] vagaries, which in my opinion were more than balanced by her energies and ability."[29]

The career of Margaret Charlton in the Faculty of Medicine of McGill University is particularly touching, and her story is one that deserves much study. She resembles other outspoken Canadian women of her period, whose colorful and dominant personalities were masked by a combination of Victorian standards and behavioral conventions. Although recognized for their work, they were frequently viewed askance by their contemporaries. Charlton's career demonstrates her success in integrating the needs of her library's users at a local level with developments in the medical library world. As she reported in 1902 to the Library Committee,

> Those engaged in research in the Library have been greatly inconvenienced by the discontinuance of the *Index Medicus*. The Index published in Paris has been found a very unsatisfactory substitute, and it seems likely to be discontinued. The Association of Medical Librarians is trying to see what can be done to start it again. I submit for your inspection for first number of the Bulletin of the Association of Medical Librarians.[30]

This quotation captures Margaret Charlton at her professional best. Her concern with adequate tools for retrieving the medical literature is clearly expressed in her dissatisfaction with the short-lived French publication, *Bibliographie Médicale*, and her efforts to improve this situation are evident. She seems in touch with her times and willing to do something to improve them. Her presentation to the Library Committee of the first volume of the *Bulletin* must have given her considerable pride. Although Charlton's career demonstrates several essential attributes of the successful librarian, we have seen that her professional life was not entirely successful. She had entered the field of medical librarianship when it was in its infancy. She appears to have lacked the management, technical, and human skills necessary in the medical librarian of today. In her defense, it is necessary to reemphasize that her profession was still being defined: the first course in medical bibliography taught by librarians was not offered until 1937, nor was there a professional librarian at the U.S. National Library of Medicine until 1942.

Osler, Gould, and Charlton—three who made an association, are shown on the Anniversary Medal struck in 1976 to commemorate the association's Seventy-fifth Annual Meeting. It depicts the three people credited with the founding of the association in 1898. On the right is the familiar, heavily moustached face of Sir William Osler, on the left, the bearded George Milbry Gould. At center, flanked by these eminent physicians, is a three-quarter profile of Margaret Charlton. Charlton's face shows a firm, even severe, expression combined with the refinement characteristic of a lady of the era. Her hair is drawn back high off her forehead, and her regular features are framed by a high Victorian collar. In sum, she appears to be very much a lady of her time.

By 1898, an association of medical librarians was an idea whose time had come. Medical education was developing rapidly in North America by the latter half of the nineteenth century, and the need for good medical libraries was increasingly evident. On May 2, 1898, George Milbry Gould invited a group of librarians to a meeting in his office at the *Philadelphia Medical Journal*, 1420 Chestnut Street, with the purpose of launching the association. Among those present were Margaret Charlton; Elizabeth Thies, librarian at the Medical and Chirurgical Faculty of Maryland; E. H. Brigham of Boston; and William Browning of Brooklyn. William Osler and J. G. Adami sent their regrets.

Although this initial meeting was an organizational one, Gould saw fit to deliver an address, "The Work of an Association of Medical Librarians." This address is in some sense predictable, demonstrating the thoughtful, righteous workings of a Civil War veteran, divinity student, and physician steeped in the literary and moral values of his time: "While war and all the forces of devolution are most active in function, it behooves those who believe in progressive evolution to do their silent and unnoticed work all the more self-sacrificingly in order that after them may live tendencies and institutions which shall make the world better."[31]

At the same time, Gould shows himself as remarkably prescient, and parts of his 1898 address could be given verbatim today:

> I look forward to such an organization of the literary [*sic*] records of medicine that a puzzled worker in any part of the civilized world shall in an hour be able to gain a knowledge pertaining to a subject from every other man in the world. It seems strange to me . . . that the pricelessly precious results of medical knowledge should be given over to the rapine of commercialism and to that barbarism of disorganization in which our medical libraries at present do not flourish. In saved lives and spared expense, our state and national governments would make money by devoting millions of dollars to establishing medical libraries in every city and village of the land. . . . Our trick seems rather to load our after-comers with debt, and to trundle our burden of all kinds upon the shoulders of the next generation.[32]

A brief chronology of events of the first five years of the association's life illustrates that the association that began in George Milbry Gould's office in May 1898 was a great success. Gould was elected the association's first president; Margaret Charlton, secretary; and Browning, treasurer. Charlton continued in this role until 1903, returning again as secretary from 1909 to 1911. The second annual meeting was also held in Philadelphia on October 5, 1899. In December of that year, the MLA Exchange was founded to be managed by Marcia Noyes. The third annual meeting of the association was held in Atlantic City in 1900, and the fourth in Baltimore in 1901 when Osler was elected the association's second president. In 1902, the fifth annual meeting took place in Saratoga Springs, New York, and Osler's presidential address was his superb essay, still in print today, "Some Aspects of American Medical Bibliography." Osler was reelected president in 1903. He was active during his presidency in encouraging physicians to join the association and send duplicates and superseded medical materials to Marcia Noyes's exchange.

In 1902, the Association of Medical Librarians began the publication of its *Bulletin of the Association of Medical Librarians*, the forerunner to the *Bulletin of the Medical Library Association* (1911–2001). During the years prior to 1911, other publications on medical libraries (*Medical Library and Historical Journal* [1903–1907] and *Medical Libraries*) existed concurrently, although the former publication was not the official record of the association. In 2002, the title was changed to *Journal of the Medical Library Association,* the current title of the official journal of record of the Medical Library Association.

Margaret Charlton welcomed the challenge of helping in the founding of the Medical Library Association and embraced these heavy responsibilities with enthusiasm. On March 31, 1898, she wrote to William

Browning, M.D., librarian of the Medical Society, County of Kings, New York: "It is proposed to form a Medical Librarians Association whereby the vast medical literature all over the world may be utilized. Dr. Gould has commissioned me to do all the correspondence relating to the formation of the Medical Librarians' Association, as he himself has not the time at present to devote to it."[33]

She continued to devote herself to this association and wrote again in May 1898 to Browning, "The more I think of our Association, the more I hope it will prove a success and that next year when we meet, it will be with the feeling that we have done our best to make it the success it deserves to be." Her dedication was sustained, but with realism evident in correspondence with Browning on June 27, 1898, "Our Library Movement seems to be growing only I think that . . . they are going a little too fast. To have a library in every village does not seem necessary."

In these early letters, Charlton also displayed her concern with some of the continuing themes in medical library practice. She was concerned that adequate collections of medical journals be established, and to this purpose wrote to publishers and medical societies to join the new association and to ask them to furnish their journals or transactions free to libraries joining the association. On the importance of separate medical libraries she wrote to Browning on July 25, 1898, "I am very much opposed to his [George M. Gould's] idea of medical libraries in public libraries and strongly maintain that medical libraries should be housed by themselves." She struck a subservient note on this issue, however, when she commented, "Of course if you . . . agree with Dr. Gould, I shall say no more about it." She was delighted to hear subsequently that Browning supported her stand in his statement: "I have read your paper which appeared in the *Philadelphia Weekly* and I am delighted with it. I agree with you in reference to the libraries being apart from general libraries wherever practical." With the second annual meeting scheduled for the autumn of 1899, Charlton was beginning to feel some pressure, revealed in her comment in a letter of October 16, 1899, to Browning, "How stupid of me to send that check . . . without endorsing it and kind of you not to say 'Just like a woman.'"

Years later in 1919, Marcia Noyes wrote to Charlton at the Academy of Medicine in Toronto, seeking clarification on the founding of the Association. In characteristic style, Charlton wrote back:

My dear Miss Noyes:
    Yes, it was my idea of starting a Medical Library Association. I do not remember if I spoke to Sir William or Dr. Gould first.
    Yours, M. Charlton.[34]

Noyes continued to be preoccupied with this question and in 1934, wrote,

> Miss Charlton was the one person who indirectly brought the Associa-
> tion into being from speaking with Dr. Osler. She had belonged to the
> American Library Association. Their problems were not our problems,
> and she felt lost and that the time was wasted, yet she had striven for
> contact with those doing just the sort of work she was doing. And so
> she suggested to Dr. Osler that it would be a fine thing if the Medical
> Librarians could do the same sort of thing the American Library Asso-
> ciation was doing.[35]

This recognition of Margaret Charlton's unique contribution to the
founding of the association is not universal. Albert Tracy Huntington takes
a somewhat different view: "The idea of forming an association of those
interested in medical libraries was conceived in the mind of one man, Dr.
George M. Gould, of Philadelphia, and he justly may be regarded as the 'father' of our Association. He presented his ideas on the subject to a few
whom he knew to be interested in medical libraries."[36]

The issue of primary recognition remains an unanswered question.
Obviously an association arose at a time when it was needed, created by devoted librarians and medical men who united in the common purpose of
improving access to medical information.

The work of Billings at the Library of the Surgeon General's Office in
establishing what was to become the U.S. National Library of Medicine and
the foundation of a speciality in medical librarianship was now in place.
Steady progress in medical librarianship was to continue, with physicians in
the leadership role. Librarians who entered this speciality took pride in an af-
filiation with physicians that distinguished them, in every sense of the word,
from other kinds of librarianship. Like physicians, medical librarians in those
early years treated their work as a vocation and were diligent in the efforts to
follow their physicians' leaders. It was not until the end of World War II that
librarian control of the Medical Library Association ended and the leadership
role of medical librarians in their association was fully established.

NOTES

1. Paul Starr, *The Social Transformation of American Medicine* (New York: Basic
Books, 1982), 15.
2. Paul Starr, *The Creation of the Media: The Political Origins of Modern Communications* (New York: Basic Books, 2004), 249.

3. Edward G. Holly, *Raking the Historic Coals* (Chicago: Beta Phi Mu, 1967), 3.

4. Estelle Brodman, *The Development of Medical Bibliography* (Chicago: Medical Library Association, 1954).

5. Wyndham D. Miles, *A History of the National Library of Medicine, the Nation's Treasury of Medical Knowledge* (Washington, DC: U.S. Public Health Service. National Institutes of Health, National Library of Medicine, 1982) (NIH Publication No. 82–1904): 18.

6. Miles, *A History of the National Library of Medicine*, 25.

7. Miles, *A History of the National Library of Medicine*, 53–55.

8. Fielding Garrison, partially unpublished memorandum in the files of the History of Medicine Division, U.S. Armed Forces Medical Library, Cleveland, Ohio, dated August 5, 1929 and quoted by Brodman, *The Development of Medical Bibliography*, 115.

9. Brodman, *The Development of Medical Bibliography*, 113.

10. John Shaw Billings, "National Catalogue of Medical Literature," quoted in Brodman, *The Development of Medical Bibliography*, 114.

11. T. E. Keyes, "Sir William Osler and the Medical Library," *Bulletin of the Medical Library Association* 49, no. 3 (January, 1961): 35.

12. Keyes, "Sir William Osler and the Medical Library," 35.

13. Harvey Cushing, *The Life of Sir William Osler*, vol. 2 (Oxford: Clarendon Press, 1925), 81.

14. A. E. Rodin and J. D. Key, "William Osler and his Persisting Textbook, 1892–1992," *Houston Med Journal* 9 (September 1993): 69–76.

15. Minnie W. Blogg, "The Johns Hopkins Hospital Library," *Bulletin of the Medical Library Association* 9, no. 1 (July, 1919): 7 (Osler Reminiscences).

16. J. Ruhräh, "Osler's Influence on Medical Libraries in America," *Bull International Assoc Med Museums J Tech Methods*, no. 9, Sir William Osler Memorial Number, *Appreciation and Reminiscences*, privately issued in Montreal, Canada, 1926: 340.

17. Cushing, *The Life of Sir William Osler*, 557.

18. Cushing, *The Life of Sir William Osler*, 625.

19. William Osler, "Books and Men," in *Aequanimitas with Other Addresses to Medical Students, Nurses and Practitioners of Medicine*, 3d ed. (Philadelphia: Blakiston, 1932), 210.

20. Osler, "Books and Men," 212.

21. William Osler, "Some Aspects of American Medical Bibliography," in *Aequanimitas with Other Addresses to Medical Students, Nurses and Practitioners of Medicine*, 3d ed. (Philadelphia: Blakiston, 1932), 299.

22. T. H. Shastid, [obituary of George Milbry Gould], *Am J Ophthalmology* 3, no. 6 (1923): 62.

23. Frances Groen, "Margaret Ridley Charlton, Medical Librarian and Historian: An Evaluation of Her Career," *Fontanus* 2 (1989): 55–63. Permission to quote from this article has been granted by president of the Management Committee of the journal.

24. W. W. Francis, "The President's Address: Margaret Charlton and the Early Days of the Medical Library Association," *Bulletin of the Medical Library Association* 25, nos. 1–2, (September, 1936): 61.

25. M. Benjamin, "The McGill Medical Library, 1829–1929," (master's thesis, McGill University, 1960), 93.

26. Francis, "The President's Address," 62.

27. The correspondence and other administrative materials related to the history of the Medical Library of McGill University are housed in the Archives of the Osler Library. The Librarian's Report and Minutes of Meetings of the Library Committee are contained in this collection. Minutes of Meetings of February 26, 1908.

28. The correspondence and other administrative materials related to the history of the Medical Library of McGill University are housed in the Archives of the Osler Library. November 29, 1912.

29. Letter from Dr. Finley to Dr. W. W. Francis, dated November 8, 1936, and quoted in Benjamin, "The McGill Medical Library," 95.

30. McGill University Faculty of Medicine, "Report of the Assistant Librarian to the Library Committee," 1902.

31. G. M. Gould, "The Work of an Association of Medical Librarians," quoted in A. T. Huntington, "The Association of Medical Librarians: Past, Present, and Future," *Bulletin of the Medical Library Association* 5 (1907): 113.

32. Gould, "The Work of an Association of Medical Librarians," 113.

33. Documents related to the history of the Medical Library Association are housed in the Archives of the National Library of Medicine, Bethesda, MD. Permission to quote from these letters is given by the executive director of the Medical Library Association. Information and quotations are drawn from Charlton's letters in this collection, dated March 31, 1898; May 6, 1898; June 27, 1898; July 18, 1898; July 25, 1898; Feb. 10, 1899; Feb. 20, 1899; May 27, 1899; July 14, 1899; Sept. 6, 1899; Sept. 19, 1899; Oct. 16, 1899; Oct. 23, 1899; and March 22, 1900.

34. Keyes, "Sir William Osler and the Medical Library," 127.

35. Marcia Noyes, "Tuesday Evening Meetings—Recorded Comments," *Bulletin of the Medical Library Association* 23 (1934): 33.

36. A. T. Huntington, "The Association of Medical Librarians: Past, Present, and Future," *Bulletin of the Medical Library Association* 5 (1907): 111.

3

THE EMERGENCE OF THE MEDICAL LIBRARY IN THE TWENTIETH CENTURY, 1900–1940

The early years of the twentieth century consolidated the innovations of the nineteenth century in the control of the medical literature and its availability to the physician. The establishment of the Association of Medical Libraries in 1898, later the Medical Library Association, with its official journal was to be a major force in the improvement of medical libraries and access to medical information. What were the priorities of the association during the early twentieth century and how did they contribute to the advancement of access to medical information? The *Bulletin*'s pages during those early years reveal a fundamental concern with the sharing of medical knowledge through the establishment of a clearinghouse for the exchange of medical publications, a desire to improve medical library operations and to control the cost of medical publications, and an abiding commitment to medical history and the medical literature of the past.

THE MEDICAL LIBRARY EXCHANGE

The establishment of the Medical Library Exchange was foremost in the minds of the founders of the association as well as its members. George Gould, as a founder of the association and a medical editor and writer, had a clear understanding of the importance of access to the literature of medicine and the value of library cooperation. The idea of exchanging medical duplicates had existed for some time. Billings had recognized its value in 1876 when he advised librarians to retain duplicate materials for completing full runs of journal titles among appropriate institutions.[1] Gould had used the pages of the *Journal of the American Medical Association* to publish lists of duplicates, launching his own exchange, but the volume of transactions and the procedures of redistribution made him more than ready to turn over this important and arduous task to the Association of Medical Libraries.

Twenty years later, the idea of the exchange remained a priority. In his presidential address to the Medical and Chirurgical Faculty of the State of Maryland in 1919,[2] John Ruhräh, who was also the editor of the *Bulletin of the Medical Library Association* along with Marcia C. Noyes, recalled the goal of establishing the exchange as a fundamental purpose of the association that Osler, Gould, and Charlton had established.

> The Association also conducts an exchange and for many years this work has been done from the Library of our Medical and Chirurgical Faculty. The Exchange distributes books, journals and reprints, taking the duplicates from the various members and distributing them among the Library members, according to several needs. The work is altruistic, the expense is paid by the Association, and the larger libraries give, while the smaller ones receive. Some idea of the scope of the work of this Association can be gained by learning that in one year they distributed about five thousand items, either books, journals, reprints or transactions to forty-three libraries.[3]

Ruhräh was a frequent contributor to the *Bulletin* and always spoke with praise about the cooperative efforts and positive results that made the Medical Library Exchange a success. One can readily appreciate why decades of medical librarians, both nationally and internationally, continued to regard the MLA Exchange as a primary benefit of membership in the Medical Library Association. The primacy of the exchange was reiterated by James F. Ballard, director of the Boston Medical Library, in an address to the Special Libraries Association in 1928:

> For thirty years the principal work of the Association has been the carrying on of the Exchange which had never ceased although its method of operation has changed from time to time. The primary membership of the Association is one of Libraries as organizations. Each member library must have at least 500 volumes. . . . The present library membership is about 110 and constantly increasing. All of the large libraries in the United States and Canada are members. The size ranges from 350,000 volumes to 700 volumes. . . . The Exchange is considered so important that a separate section in the By-Laws has to do with provisions for its management.[4]

One of the chief benefits of association membership was participation in the exchange, an outstanding example of early cooperative initiatives in the library field. Libraries were given precedence in the disposal of material available through the exchange, based upon their size, the largest library being first. Prioritizing libraries according to their size recognized that larger libraries purchased more and therefore needed less material from the exchange since most of what they needed had already been purchased. Large libraries also had more duplicate volumes to contribute to the exchange. The manager of the exchange compiled lists of duplicate materials for distribution to member libraries. The exchange acted as a clearinghouse for requests for materials, coordinating the needs and matching these to the providers. The volumes were shipped by the owner directly to the requestor. This practical process avoided the problem of the accumulation of duplicate materials at a central depot, a practice on which many book exchange programs have floundered. A provision was made to store materials only if materials could not be retained due to space problems. The exchange remained at the very heart of the association's activities. Over the years, efforts continued to improve the efficiency and cost effectiveness of the exchange, encouraging prompt delivery of requested items and prompt return of requests to the exchange. Many years later in the late 1990s, when the future of the exchange was under consideration for budgetary problems, the membership of the Medical Library Association gave an outstanding endorsement of its importance to the community

THE GREAT WAR, 1914–1918

During the first year of World War I, three years prior to the entry of the United States in 1917, an unsigned editorial in the *Bulletin* reflected the negative impact of the European war on the availability of the medical publications:

> All the French publications have been suspended with the exception of *Presse Médicale*, which has been reduced to a four-page bulletin. . . . The Belgian journals, naturally, have ceased altogether, although they kept up a little longer than the French. The Italian journals have suffered more than would seem to be necessary. . . . The German journals have been delayed considerably . . . the Austrian journals have either been suspended since the middle of August or have not arrived for reasons of transportation.[5]

The author continues in this vein, commenting upon the suspension of medical research in war time, the curtailment of work in the universities and a refocusing of priorities on military medicine. The conclusion predicts a reduction in European medical publishing, resulting from the conflagrations.

Three years later in the pages of this same journal, the lead article, signed "F. H. G." (Fielding H. Garrison), provides a more dramatic description of the medical library at war:

> Books have been described as "highly explosive compounds," products of the diabolical, cerebral chemistry of authors. Printers are munition workers, publishing houses munition plants, and libraries are arsenals where the dangerous ordnance stores are arranged in rows. Shall we define the Librarians as the "bronze artillery officer" who directs his assistants to send them to their destination—with the poor bibliographers as a range-finder?[6]

F. H. G. continues in marshalling the medical librarian to war, insisting that the medical librarian can certainly "do his bit" . . . by simply bringing his munition stores to the front for immediate use. Numerous basic military manuals and handbooks are identified, and in the commitment of medical librarians to preserve the medical past, F. H. G. describes an imaginary exhibit of military medical classics. The imaginary exhibit includes Gersdorf and Fabricius Hildanus on military surgery, Ambroise Paré and John Hunter on gunshot wounds, and works on military hospitals, military hygiene, as well as "a relief from a Babylonian state representing a battlefield with vultures as scavengers, collection of the wounded and burial of the dead in a common pit."[7]

At the same time, Grace W. Myers, librarian of the Massachusetts General Hospital Treadwell Library, was concerned with bibliographic access, in particular, appropriate subject classification of materials on warfare and surgical and base hospitals units, and the retrieval of medical material related to the war. Her introduction to the question of war bibliography resonates with the same emotional commitment as F. H. G:

> In these strenuous times, when the heart of every true American is stirred to its depths and each individual be he soldier or civilian, is spurred on to his very best efforts for the sake of country, it behooves us librarians to search our shelves for what is needed to meet the emergency. The dark clouds of war draw closer about us, and the Medical Department of our Army is calling to its ranks many physicians and sur-

geons whose faces are familiar to our reading rooms and whose friendly greetings we are bound to miss. What are we doing for them?[8]

The editorial by F. H. G. and the article by Grace Myers capture the founding priorities of access to information and preservation of the past that continue as priorities of the medical library community.

One month before the 1918 armistice, another unsigned editorial describes "difficulties due to the war." The association had decided not to hold an annual meeting in 1918, with the result that the amount of materials available for publication was curtailed. It is noted that "the Exchange is holding its own, in spite of the difficulties under which shipping is done." In a note following, a further war supporting initiative is announced to readers of the *Bulletin*: "All our members have been in receipt of notifications from the publishers of journals which have been sent to them complimentary, stating that under the ruling of the War Industries Board it was recommended that they discontinue sending out free journals as a means of economizing paper."[9]

Receiving European publications and, for medical libraries, German publications in particular, was a concern. The American Library Association was of assistance in helping all libraries in this area of foreign acquisitions during this period as recorded in the pages of the *Bulletin*:

> Few Medical Libraries received any German periodicals after the beginning of 1916, although most of us subscribed through our chosen agents for 1916 and 1917, many ordering that these be held abroad until cessation of hostilities. After America's entry into the war, in the spring of 1917, complications arose which made it seem a forlorn hope. In 1918 arrangements were made by the American Library Association with the State Department and the War Trade and Censorship Boards, in Washington, for the importation of a limited number of journals by institutions.[10]

STOCKING THE SHELVES

Following the end of the war, libraries enjoyed a return to normalcy, a period of reasonable growth and stability of funding. Science, business, and professionalism were rewarded. However, by the late 1920s, medical libraries had identified two major areas of concern that threatened their ability to fulfill their commitment to providing access to information: the tools for bibliographic access and control of the medical literature were complex, incomplete, and frequently not timely, with a series of overlapping indexes and catalogs.[11] And the prices of journals were too high.

There were also concerns with the coverage, or rather the lack of coverage, of medical journals in the only English-language index, the *Quarterly Cumulative Index Medicus*. Librarians recognized that a journal that was not indexed may as well not have been written. The tension between access to "the best" writing as opposed to comprehensive coverage of the literature resonates to the present day in discussions regarding what is appropriate for inclusion in the MEDLINE database.

By far the most important concern and one that continues to the present, was the high cost of the journal literature. Early dialog between medical librarians and publishers is reflected in this short note from a roundtable discussion held during the meeting of the Medical Library Association:

> We have continued a friendly correspondence with the German publishers and beg to report that favorable changes may be made in the near future. Mr. Springer has promised us at the end of this year a list of his journals with the number of volumes to appear in 1928 and their approximate cost. He advises us that it will show a reduction in output due to his efforts in having articles written in briefer form and having caught up with previously accepted manuscript [sic].[12]

Mr. Springer's news must have been well received, especially on the eve of the Great Depression.

North American medical librarians were hard pressed to continue to provide journal access to their users. Hammered by the Great Depression that cut their budgets and annual, unpredictable costly increases in journal subscriptions, medical librarians began to study the problem. German periodicals were particularly problematic, and, during this period, the German language was as important as English in scientific and medical communication. A particularly informative study was done at the Library of the College of Physicians and Surgeons of Columbia University by Alfred Robert.[13] Robert's paper is one of the earliest and most comprehensive in a series of studies that continue into the present electronic environment. It was based on the journals received in the College of Physicians and Surgeons Library during 1930–1931 and had, as its basic purpose "an attempt to ascertain the cause of yearly deficits in the budget, which always occurred in the appropriations for subscriptions to periodicals." The particular concern was the cost of German medical periodicals and the failure of the German publishers to establish fixed annual subscription rates and to regulate annual production. The fact that German publishers were issuing so many supplementary volumes each year in the form of Festschriften, Beiheft, and so on was identified as a further contributing factor to the high costs of the German medical periodical literature. A careful analysis of the journals received in the library from domestic, British, French, and German publishers analyzed the cost per page of the journals. The results were most revealing, showing that expenditures on German periodicals were five times that spent on American publications, eight times the dollars spent on British, and sixteen times the amount spent on publications that originated in France. The authors conclude with a series of reasonable recommendations to the German publishing industry, including the need for a fixed annual subscription price, restrictions on supplementary volumes, and a reduction in the total amount of material to be published by at least 30 percent. Many of these same issues resurface in a more complex, collaborative, and agitated environment at the end of the twentieth century in the electronic journal era. The most significant change is that German is no longer a primary language of international medical communication.

Fielding H. Garrison, who had left the Library of the Office of the Surgeon General for the Welch Medical Library at Johns Hopkins also took up the issue of journal costs.[14] Garrison did not take on the task of bibliometric analysis. He comments on the fact that German medical publishers pay their authors, but, as pointed out by Robert, fail to provide a precise annual subscription rate and charge significantly for supplementary volumes. Garrison is at pains to stress the very high quality of German titles such as *Hoppe-Seyler's Zeitschrift* and the massive amount of material contained in *Biochemische Zeitschrift*, which by 1930 included fourteen volumes for that year alone. He identifies a number of German periodicals, concluding that they are unable to compete with their American counterparts and draws the resounding conclusion that "the articles in the periodical literature of recent German medicine are extraordinarily lengthy, prolix, and verbose and about this matter, the best type of German savant will make merry on occasion if you can draw him out."[15]

A Committee on Costs of Current Medical Periodicals had been established as a priority by the Medical Library Association, and was chaired by Eileen R. Cunningham of Vanderbilt University. Cunningham's committee continued to provide substantial reports on the issue of journal pricing throughout the 1930s. It found that approximately two-thirds of the annual budget for journals in medical libraries in North America was being spent on periodicals of German origin.[16] The medical librarians were not alone in their concerns, as medical scientists in both the United States and elsewhere became aware of these issues through the work of the association. A ground swell of concern resulted in a resolution by the membership at its meeting in 1933 in Baltimore that after December 1934, the budgets of medical libraries would not maintain subscriptions to journals that cost more then forty dollars per year. This resolution drew a line in the sand of accounting, and there followed what appears to have been discussions and promises from publishers that failed to show results. The medical librarians acting in the public interest finally achieved results when a group of German scientific publishers agreed to reduce the size and price of selected publications by 20 percent, but the necessary implementation did not occur. Further discussion resulted in the arrival of the director of Verlag Chemie and Julius Springer in Chicago, participating in discussions with librarians during a meeting of the American Library Association. A reasonable compromise was, at least for the time being, arrived at when Julius Springer proposed a 30-percent reduction in some of its most expensive medical titles, as well as a subsequent offer to reduce further the costs of Springer titles. Evidently, Springer delivered on its promises, although, as we shall show throughout this work, constant vigilance on the subject of the costs of periodicals remained a matter of priority for medical librarians. The work of medical librarians on behalf of the community of medical and scientific users received the appreciation of the Federation of American Societies for Experimental Biology. Other societies, among them the American Physiological Society, the American Society of Biological Chemists, and the American Society for Pharmacology and Experimental Therapeutics, joined in expressing their gratitude and encouragement for the continuing efforts of the medical librarians. For the moment, Alfred Robert and Eileen Cunningham had set a high level of effectiveness in controlling the costs of medical journals, thereby ensuring, at least for the time being, access to the medical journal literature.

Selection and costs of medical periodicals are at the heart of the activities of medical libraries. In 1934, R. L. Jenkins, a physician, provided readers of the *Bulletin* with an interesting approach to the selection of medical periodicals.[17] Jenkins analyzed the references that appeared in the *Journal of the American Medical Association*, the *British Medical Journal*, and the *Klinische Wochenschrift*. To be considered desirable, each journal required at least three citations in the journals cited by articles in these periodicals, and these journals were weighted by frequency of citation and by cost. Jenkins shared this information with Eileen Cunningham. The careful analysis of journals and their selection as well as their cost continued to preoccupy medical librarians throughout the decade.

Cunningham continued to study the matter, with special attention to the pricing of the twenty-six journals for which Springer had agreed to reduce prices. Again, through her chairing of the Medical Library Association's Committee on the Cost of Current Medical Periodicals, she reported in the pages of the *Bulletin* regarding the crisis faced by medical librarians in the publication of medical and biological literature. Studies of journal pricing were proliferating, an increasing number of journals were being published, library budgets were declining in the time of the Depression, and librarians were increasingly critical. With insight and foresight, she hits the nail on the head by raising a fundamental question, one that the librarians and academic communities have yet to respond to.

> Does all of the mass of published literature represent *chiefly* the result of investigative data concerning fundamental discoveries? It is regrettable that the answer must be *no*. Unquestionably other factors have entered in, and certain of them seem of particular importance. In some countries institutional appointments and promotions have been to a certain extent dependent upon the number of titles that are included in a candidate's bibliography. The natural result has been to split papers into more and more units.[18]

She called for the leaders in education to emphasize content and quality rather than the number of titles and articles that are published, and in doing so walked down a path generations must continue to tread until the issue is fully addressed. As always, her conclusions are balanced, recognizing the legitimate reasons for the increasing amounts of medical information being published, while recognizing that there exists an increasing tendency to publish unnecessary material. Her conclusion echoes over time to support the idea of open access, discussed in detail later in this book.

> The problem is not a simple one, and numerous difficulties lie in the path of its satisfactory solution; nevertheless, the solution is of great importance because it seems certain that, unless the entire field of publication in the medical and allied sciences is placed on as noncommercial a basis as possible, radical and perhaps regrettable changes are inevitable.[19]

In subsequent reports, Cunningham looks at the technical and organizational responses to the problem of escalating journal costs, proposing the use of photographic technology and a central, cooperative organization that would act in the public good by providing bibliographies and copies of the current and retrospective articles. Unless these issues were addressed, she foresaw an ever increasing dilemma for future generations of medical librarians, as well as clinicians and researchers. She called for cooperation and "the setting aside of individual jealousies and prejudices" if the present situation is to change.[20]

MEDICAL HISTORY AND MEDICAL LIBRARIANSHIP

The association, as we have seen, was founded by doctors and one librarian, and the librarian founder, Margaret Charlton, never served as president of the association she had helped to launch. The other founders did; George M. Gould was founding president in 1898 and Sir William Osler became president for the first time in 1901. This preponderance of physicians, especially a bibliographer and medical historian such as Osler and an editor and author such as Gould, played a role in fostering a strong interest on the part of medical librarians and physicians alike in medical history. The large number of articles on historical topics that were published in the *Bulletin* prior to the Second World War gives ample evidence of this interest. Medical librarians as well as physicians authored numerous historical publications. The American Association for the History of Medicine had been founded in 1925, but despite its existence, there was no diminution in articles on medical history published in the *Bulletin*. Doubtlessly, the knowledge and enthusiasm of William Osler encouraged medical librarians in Canada, England, and the United States to develop an interest in medical history. As a result, the medical historical library legacy is a very strong one, and the preservation of the accumulated wisdom of the past is a core value of the profession of medical librarianship, in part due to the work of the early leaders in the field.

Margaret Charlton, one of the founders of the association, had herself been a serious student of medical history, publishing a series of articles on the subject of early medicine in Lower Canada (Québec).[21] We have no record of her reasons for choosing to publish this quite extensive series of articles in the *Annals* rather than in the official publication of the association that she had founded. We do know that, despite her nineteen years as head of the Medical Library of McGill University, Montreal, she did not return to the McGill campus to celebrate with members of the Medical Library Association the arrival of Osler's Library in the Faculty of Medicine. W. W. Francis, Osler's nephew, who arrived with Osler's books at McGill as Osler Librarian, speculated on the unhappiness that surrounded Charlton's departure from McGill University in 1914. He notes somewhat poignantly in his President's Address that

> to lose a job to which one has devoted head, heart, hand and twenty of one's best years must be one of the major tragedies of life. . . . Her

principles, I think, were uncompromisingly rigid. For years she had worked happily under a chief, the Honorary Librarian, a member of the faculty, one who is an extraordinarily angelic combination of wisdom, courtesy, patience and good humor. . . . In 1913 he was succeeded by a new broom which raised a lot of dust. . . . The irresistible force met an immovable spirit in a not quite immovable body, and in May, 1915, she resigned. A bitter sense of injustice prevented her ever revisiting her old haunts, and 15 years later I could not induce her to come open or surreptitiously, to see the newly arrived Osler Library which would have interested her intensely.[22]

Dr. W. W. Francis served as the twenty-third president of the Medical Library Association (1935) and Osler Librarian. Like Osler, he fostered an interest in medical history through his curatorship of the eight thousand rare medical volumes that Osler had bequeathed to McGill. Medical history was a compelling interest to many medical librarians who heard his address "At Osler's Shrine" at the annual meeting of the Medical Library Association in Richmond in May 1937, where he expanded on the gloriously rich life of Osler.[23] Osler was indeed enshrined in the hearts and minds of librarians and physicians, as Francis's address indicates.

This interest in medical history by the medical library profession has helped to foster a commitment to the preservation of the medical past. The hagiography that was captured in Francis's title of his 1937 address, "At Osler's Shrine," cannot go unnoticed. The study of the history of medicine was to mature in later years, and move away from the story of great physicians and to raise new questions regarding the traditional relationship between patients and physicians. The iconography of a medical history based on the study of the great men of medicine was to undergo considerable revision by the end of the century. Richard Horton, physician, medical writer, and editor of the *Lancet*, has, in our own time, provided librarians, physicians, and all readers interested in health care with a fresh version of Sir William, the man and the myth. Medical science in the early twenty-first century has been redefined to include the global burden of disease, genetic modification, and human genome research. Matters that once were the exclusive purview of the physician have become matters of public concern. On the topic of Osler, Horton provides a balance between respect and the need to move away from the shrine:

> There is much in Osler's life to study with modern advantage. His achievements are a remarkable testament to professional ideals that deserve discussion and reinterpretation among every new generation of medical practitioners. But to sustain the Osler myth, as doctors and

medical historians have done, serves only to promote a version of medicine that is disengaged both from contemporary clinical inquiry and the difficult political discussions that affect the future of health care. These enquiries and debates need fresh thinking, not curatorial reverence.[24]

By the 1930s, the collaboration between the U.S. Surgeon General's Office and the Medical Library Association was in full flower. Congress had approved the construction of the new Army Medical Library in early 1938, and a bill for its creation had been signed by the president in June 1938. Thoughts of a much-needed new building were prominent in the minds of many medical librarians, including a special consideration for the history of medicine.[25] In the new library the world catalog of medical books would continue, and a book binding department would be part of the new facility. There was even some speculation during this planning period regarding the establishment of a school for medical librarians or some form of training at a postgraduate level in the specialty of medical librarianship, medical bibliography, and medical history. The future of the *Index-Catalogue* was also under review, since the production of annual citations had grown to 120,000 references per year, and the Government Printing Office was working at maximum capacity. The Library of the Office of the Surgeon General was over a century old, and its present, totally inadequate facilities were more than fifty years old. Growth of the national collection and developments in medical librarianship had rendered a new facility an absolute necessity. Unfortunately, events were unfolding in Europe that would have serious implications for governments and their priorities.

The Medical Library Association had reached its fortieth birthday in 1938 and the president that year, James Ballard, reflected on its history and its current challenges.[26] Responsible fiscal management and cost effectiveness were major considerations. The issues of the costs of the journal literature continued as a matter of priority for all medial librarians. Ballard was pleased to report that the scope of the Committee on Periodicals and Serials of the Medical Library Association had broadened to consider all of the problems related to the acquisition of periodicals. It had achieved a discount of 25 percent and the "limitation and standardization of the number of volumes published each year has been the direct result of the campaign against excessive costs."[27] Outreach was also a continuing concern, as medical librarians increasingly recognized the value of collaboration outside their own specialization. In 1935, the association had joined the International Federation of Library Associations (IFLA) to promote international library cooperation.

By 1939, Europe was again at war and, although the United States would not enter for more than two years, North American medical librarians were beginning to feel the impact. One aspect was the difficulty experienced by its Committee on Periodicals and Serials in completing the annual comparative study on the yearly costs of German medical periodicals, due to the delayed receipt of foreign journals in the United States. The impact of the war in Europe was beginning to be felt in the nature and production of scientific publications. Journals would cease publications and mail service would be suspended. International collaboration on journal pricing among libraries would reach a standstill.

At a more fundamental level, transcending particular professional issues and journal publication, was the alarm, largely unheeded, that rings too clearly today. In an article on foreign medical directories, this brief, chilling, factual note describing the contents of *Verzeichnis der Deutschen Ärzte und Heilanstalten* for 1937 occurs:

> Revised biennially. Supplements issued frequently. Alphabetical and geographical registered are included with Jewish physicians indicated with special symbols. . . . Communication from publisher (1938) stated that an index for Austria was not expected. . . . In June, 1939 it was understood at the American Consulate in Vienna that the Austrian names would be included in the 1940 directory.[28]

NOTES

1. Jennifer Connor, *Guardians of Medical Knowledge:The Genesis of the Medical Library Association* (Lanham, MD: Medical Library Association and Scarecrow Press, 2000), 44.

2. John Ruhräh, "The Medical Library" (presidential address delivered before the Medical and Chirurgical Faculty of the State of Maryland, April 22, 1919), *Bulletin of the Medical Library Association* 8, no. 4 (April, 1919): 41–50.

3. Ruhräh, "The Medical Library," 49.

4. James F. Ballard, "The Medical Library Exchange," *Bulletin of the Medical Library Association* 17, no. 4 (October 1928): 36.

5. "The War and Medical Literature," *Bulletin of the Medical Library Association* 4, no. 2 (October 1914): 28.

6. F. H. G., "The Medical Library in Wartime" [editorial], *Bulletin of the Medical Library Association* 7, no. 2 (October 1917): 29–32.

7. F. H. G., "The Medical Library in Wartime," 32.

8. Grace W. Myers, "War Bibliography," *Bulletin of the Medical Library Association* 7, no. 2 (October 1917): 25–27.

9. "Difficulties Due to the War: Free Journals for Librarians" [unsigned], *Bulletin of the Medical Library Association* 8, no. 2 (October, 1918): 27–28.

10. "German Periodicals for 1919" [unsigned], *Bulletin of the Medical Library Association* 8, no. 2 (1918): 28.

11. The following bibliographies were required for accessing the medical literature: (1) *Index Catalogues* of the Library of the Surgeon General's Office.

1st series, 1880–1895

2nd series, 1896–1916

3rd series, 1916–1932

4th series, 1936–

(2) *Quarterly Cumulative Index to Current Medical Literature.* Published by the American Medical Association, semiannual publication beginning in 1916–1926, covering the same field as *Index Medicus* for the period.

Index Medicus, three series.

1st 1879–1899

2nd 1903–1920

3rd 1921–1927

Contained material not found in the *Index Catalogue.*

In 1926, the *Index Medicus* and the *Quarterly Cumulative Index Medicus* combined. For the period, 1900–1902, medical librarians relied largely upon the French publication *Bibliographie Médicale*, 1900–1902, 3 vols., edited by Marcel Baudouin.

12. *Bulletin of the Medical Library Association* 17, no. 4. (December 1928): 41.

13. Alfred L. Robert and Hans H. Schallenbrand, "The Comparative Cost of Medical Journals," *Bulletin of the Medical Library Association* 20, no. 4 (April 1932): 140–53.

14. Fielding Garrison, "The High Cost of Current Medical Periodicals," *Bulletin of the Medical Library Association* 20, no. 4 (April 1932): 165–69.

15. Garrison, "The High Cost of Current Medical Periodicals," 169.

16. "Report of the Committee on the Cost of Current Medical Periodicals for the Year 1933–1934," *Bulletin of the Medical Library Association* 23, no. 1 (August 1934): 36.

17. R. L. Jenkins, "Cost Analysis of Medical Periodicals," *Bulletin of the Medical Library Association* 22, no. 3 (January 1934): 115.

18. Eileen R. Cunningham, "The Present Status of the Publication of Literature in the Medical and Biological Sciences," *Bulletin of the Medical Library Association* 24, no. 1 (August 1934): 66.

19. Cunningham, "The Present Status," 73.

20. Eileen R. Cunningham, "Looking Forward: Possible Developments in the Publication of Medical Literature," *Bulletin of the Medical Library Association* 25, nos. 1–2 (September 1936): 100–108.

21. Margaret Charlton, "Outlines of the History of Medicine in Lower Canada," *Annals of Medical History* 5 (1923): 150–74, 263–78; 6 (1924): 222–35, 312–54.

22. W. W. Francis, "The President's Address: Margaret Charlton and the Early Days of the Medical Library Association" (read at the annual dinner of the Medical Library Association, St. Paul, Minnesota, June 22, 1936), *Bulletin of the Medical Library Association* 25, nos. 1–2 (September 1936): 59.

23. Francis, "The President's Address: At Osler's Shrine," *Bulletin of the Medical Library Association* 26, nos. 1–2 (October 1937): 1–9.

24. Richard Horton, *Health Wars: On the Global Front Lines of Modern Medicine* (New York: New York Review of Books, 2004), 247.

25. Harold Wellington Jones, "Some Thoughts on the Future of the Army Medical Library," *Bulletin of the Medical Library Association* 27 no. 1 (October 1938): 32–34.

26. James F. Ballard, "The President's Address" (given at the annual meeting of the Medical Library Association, Boston, MA, June 25, 1938), *Bulletin of the Medical Library Association* 27, no. 1 (October 1938): 1–17.

27. Ballard, "President's Address," 11.

28. "A Checklist of Foreign Medical Directories of the Medical and Some Allied Professions, 1930–1940," compiled by Irene Macy Strieby, *Bulletin of the Medical Library Association* 28, no. 4 (June 1940): 210.

4

THE WAR AND AFTER, 1940–1960

In the previous chapter, the strong relationship between physicians, the history of medicine, and medical librarians was noted. A review of the pages of the *Bulletin of the Medical Library Association* demonstrates this emphasis on the past: the war years appear to have given rise to an outflow of interest in medical history. In the four issues of *Bulletin of the Medical Library Association* for 1944, a total of thirty-one articles were published, excluding regular features such as "Association News," "Committee Reports," and editorials. Of those thirty-one articles, twenty-one were on topics of medical history. This is not to say that the published record of medical librarianship demonstrated a lack of concern with the present realities of the war and the need to plan for postwar recovery. Rather, the harsh realities of the war left little time and fewer dollars for innovation and growth in medical libraries. As the war was drawing to an end, there was a strong desire to turn away from those dark years and to address issues that had, of necessity, been preempted in order to support the war effort. This resurgence of hope was highly evident, and it was to have an enormous effect on all libraries, and most particularly, the U.S. National Library of Medicine. The year before the end of hostilities, Harold Wellington Jones, director of the Army Medical Library from 1936 to 1945, captured this spirit, "The Army Medical Library is emerging from its long sleep. It is attempting to organize for the immediate future as the greatest medical library in the world."[1]

Early in the war, medical librarians demonstrated their commitment to serving military physicians, using a form of regionalization to supply as many services as possible at a local level, an approach that today still characterizes library cooperation and consorted activity. Looking to the role of medical librarians after the end of hostilities, in an editorial Mary Louise Marshall[2] called on medical librarians to be prepared for the influx of returning service personnel who would be taking advantage of the postwar educational opportunities provided by the government. Librarians could assist through the provision of library resources and facilities. Speculation on the nature of a new national medical library that had to be put on hold during the war years was to be reinvigorated, as a priority, during the postwar period. This speculation included the relationship between a new national library and the Library of Congress. The location of this new library was also debated. Proximity to the offices of the American Medical Association in Chicago was thought in some quarters to be desirable. And what would be the relationship between this library and other major medical libraries that had grown up in universities and academies around the country? But before these questions that had been put on hold in 1941 could be addressed, those concerned with the future development of medical libraries and information had to pass through the war years.

The war created two major challenges for librarians: the incompleteness of library holdings as a result of lost materials and, in Europe, the actual destruction of libraries. The former, a challenge of identifying full runs of the journal literature, was addressed by the compilation of union lists of foreign periodicals in all disciplines. Eventually a copy of a missing journal was usually located in a library in the United States or Canada. The effort of North American and British librarians to maintain comprehensive library collections is captured in a letter to the *Bulletin of the Medical Library Association* from Leslie Morton, then the librarian at the St. Thomas Hospital Medical School, Guildford, Surrey, where the school had been relocated from London in 1941 to protect it from Nazi bombings. Morton expresses his appreciation to North American librarians for their assistance in completing journal runs, but notes, in a fine spirit of cooperation, and despite the challenges facing British librarians at this point, that British librarians would like to assist their North American counterparts in the same manner:

> While thanking you for your kindness in helping to replace these gaps, I feel that the English libraries should, as far as possible, reciprocate by collecting here any journals lost by American medical libraries. If the Association has any idea of the extent of such losses perhaps you would be kind enough to let me know, and I will see if anything can be arranged. As you know, we have no Association devoted solely to medical librarians, but if nothing has yet been done, I am sure that with the help of C.C. Barnard of the London School of Hygiene, I might be able to collect the greater part of what is wanted by medical libraries in the U.S.A.[3]

The destruction of entire libraries in Europe is a devastation of which even today the cultural implications cannot be fully understood. In the Soviet Union, for example, it was estimated that seventeen million volumes were lost.[4] This was a moment for librarians to reflect on their core values of providing access to information and preserving the cultural and intellectual heritage. The time was now for the assertion of the importance of libraries as essential in the recovery of a war torn world. The devastation of the war provided a unique opportunity to rebuild, to reconceptualize the nature of the library, and to reassert the importance of library cooperation. Information technology to advance access to information was not yet developed, with the exception of microfilming, but library cooperation, at both a national and international level, appeared to be the single most viable way to solve the problems of libraries in the immediate postwar era.

Regular practice and procedures in medical libraries felt the impact of the war in Europe. Just as during the First World War there was a need to expand the subject retrieval system to deal with military medical practice, so again, medical librarians looked to improve their management of military information. Since the outbreak of hostilities in 1939, the pertinent literature had experienced considerable growth. The concept of "military medicine" expanded to include civilian populations who were part of air raids. Based on her experience in handling these materials in the Library of the Vanderbilt University School of Medicine, Eileen Cunningham again came forward, this time to provide a revised subject classification in order to serve this purpose.[5] The same issue of the *Bulletin of the Medical Library Association* that contains Cunningham's revised subject classification contains a full listing of materials on war medicine[6] and notes that these materials may be borrowed from the Army Medical Library.

During the war years, the "Foreign News" column in the *Bulletin of the Medical Library Association* provided a forum for the communication of problems and needs between European librarians, mainly British, and North American medical librarians. The letters published in this recurring feature of the *Bulletin* tell repeatedly stories of medical library disasters, near disasters, and needs. They reveal a strong sense of mutual concern that extended between medical librarians on both sides of the Atlantic. These brief communications must have made the war experience vivid to the more protected librarians of North America in, for example, the inclusion of information snippets such as,

> Food is so scarce in occupied Poland that people have to eat their domestic animals. A pound of dog meat costs $1.78, and a cat sells for

$4.45, skin and bones included. In France, conditions are not much better, and a French food manufacturing company (of all things) began to advertise a miraculous substance to kill appetite. A teaspoonful of this substance is sufficient to make anyone satiated even on a meager diet.[7]

Devastation through war was a constant threat to libraries. But a second concern was the repression of information, in the spirit of the wartime adage, "a slip of the lip might sink a ship." In this area, a letter from the librarian of King's College Library, Newcastle-on-Tyne, written in November 1942, documents the subsidiary concern.

> One further matter I should like to mention. The September 1942 number of the *American Journal of Medical Sciences* arrived here with an article deleted by the censor. This presumably applies to all copies imported into this country, and while evidently no replacement of this imperfect part is possible during the war, perfect copies will be wanted after the war and will be most valuable. I hope they may be collected and treasured by your Association until the happy time when they can be shipped to this country.[8]

The American Library Association with the help of the Rockefeller Foundation undertook the task of prioritizing scientific and technical periodicals for war-ravaged libraries in Europe and the Far East. The purpose was to guarantee the presence of at least one set of an important title for each country. By the time the war ended, a large, at times confusing, array of organizations and institutions were concerned with assistance to libraries. Considerable coordination of effort was needed. Perhaps prematurely, the Library of Congress had convened a conference on this issue, with a limited number of fifty invitees, due to wartime restrictions on travel. One positive outcome was the creation of a Joint Committee on Books for Devastated and Other Libraries with the support of the U.S. Department of State, the Library of Congress, and other agencies.[9] The importance of cooperation at the international level could not be overemphasized.

It was difficult to comprehend the magnitude of damage to foreign medical literature. What publications had been suspended, what ones had ceased, what issues had never been sent, although published, the devastation of foreign book centers, especially the large German ones in Berlin and Leipzig—all of these issues were addressed by the Committee on Periodicals and Serial Publications of the Medical Library Association so capably chaired by Eileen R. Cunningham. She had already done great service to the medical library community through her work in the 1930s in documenting serial price increases and in advocating for limiting cost, as described in chapter 3. She served all librarians well as the representative of the Medical Library Association on the Joint Committee on Importation of the American Library Association, the Medical Library Association, and the Special Libraries Association.

In North America, medical librarians could look forward to advancing their efforts, but in Europe, the devastation of the war created a different dynamic. The losses faced by European libraries must have seemed insurmountable. At least one British medical librarian found the time to comment on this period in the pages of the *Bulletin*:

> As part of the price the nations have had to pay for becoming embroiled in another great war, the world is poorer by, it is estimated, some 5 million books and documents, as a result of military operations. As early as October 1941 Viscount Samuel stated in the House of Lords that already 20 million volumes had been destroyed in libraries public and private, in Britain. These figures include the six million books in publishers' stocks which were reduced to ashes in the heavy raids on London in May, 1941.[10]

The intensity of the Luftwaffe blitz on London had resulted in damage to a number of libraries with culturally significant holdings, including the British Museum, which lost one hundred fifty thousand volumes in one night, University College, King's College, and the Guildhall Library. But according to Wigmore, medical libraries, by chance, had been spared such massive devastation. Some libraries were evacuated for safekeeping, such as the Royal Society of Medicine, which was evacuated to Hertfordshire in the country with the aid of the Rockefeller Foundation. Despite a direct hit, the Library of the Royal College of Surgeons remained reasonably unscathed as well, although windows were blown out and the ceilings collapsed. This library, too, had evacuated some of its most valuable items to the National Library of Wales. What is called "disaster planning" in today's libraries was well established, as seen in the plans of the London School of Hygiene and Tropical Medicine made prior to the outbreak of hostilities to evacuate the most valuable parts of the collection to Tunbridge Wells, Kent. The Library of the Royal College of Physicians, like that of the Royal College of Surgeons, was similarly blessed when, despite a blast that was strong enough to hurl books from their shelves, there was relatively minor damage to the books themselves, which were removed just before a heavy rain began to fall on the bomb site. Such stories of loss and loss prevented are more than charming anecdotes. They tell of the fragility of our cultural heritage and of the determination of librarians to preserve and defend that heritage.

The situation in continental Europe was, of course, more devastating, as looting by occupying armies also played a role in the devastation of great libraries. It is difficult to separate the medical collection loss from the general book theft and destruction, since many of the great libraries of Europe were both science and humanities collections. Wigmore documents the loss of three million books in five Polish universities.[11] Nazi strategy in the occupied territories was also one of humiliation in the occupied country. Destruction of symbols of cultural heritage, such as books and libraries, served as an instrument of control, and eliminated cultural artifacts as symbols of the history of the occupied country. Some damage was irreparable, but there was much that could be done when hostilities ended to repair the damage. The need to rebuild provided an opportunity for meaningful and productive contact between librarians in North America and Europe to organize cooperative efforts in rebuilding libraries. The importance of the work of the American Library Association's Committee on Devastated Libraries and its successor, the Committee on Aid to Libraries in War Areas, and the financial support of the Rockefeller Foundation during the reconstruction period deserves special commendation.

The war and its aftermath created the need for medical librarians to review and develop their programs in a number of areas. The medical school curriculum was under revision and librarians needed to adapt to changes in medical education. The nature and content of reference work, the need for improved funding, or at least, a return of funding that had been reduced in the interest of the war effort, required new solutions, ones that would be found through imagining new futures for the medical library and the delivery of medical information. A new emphasis on timeliness in the delivery of medical information, both in relation to patient care and in research, had emerged during the war years. Extended service—service on demand—had become part of the war effort, and expectations had been raised. The "banking hours" that had existed in some libraries in the prewar era were no longer tolerable in an era where access to information ceased when the library closed. The war had created the need for library staff to improve quality in the acquisition, processing, and delivery of medical and scientific information, and the question of education and training in medical librarianship emerged as a major issue in the years following the end of the war. As army medical personnel returned to school and to civilian life, reform of the medical curriculum necessitated new library initiatives and, in some instances, especially in the case of the U.S. National Library of Medicine, new library services at a national level.

Medical librarians in North America had chosen not to hold meetings of the Medical Library Association during the war years, 1942–1945. They were, however, both active and productive during this period, although the stimulation of the personal contact provided by an annual meeting was absent. One of the most productive and long-lasting initiatives, which continues to the present, was the appearance in 1943 of the *Handbook of Medical Library Practice*. The first postwar meeting of the association, held in New Haven in 1946, emphasized the importance of training and certification for medical librarianship. The war years had indeed created new opportunities and professional needs, and the medical librarian community was prepared to establish standards of practice in the interests of providing excellence in medical information delivery.

Mildred Jordan described certification for medical librarianship as the second stage of professionalization, the first being the founding of a professional association.[12] A profession is fundamentally a group of individuals organized to meet a social need, and both in the founding of the association and in the development of training and certification programs, medical librarians had responded to this social need. Professional standards evolve as a means of guaranteeing that the public receives an appropriate level of service and quality. These actions served to maintain standards and at the same time to advance the status of the librarian as a professional practitioner. The programs needed to ensure standards of practice in medical librarianship were intensely debated. Medical librarian certification was, from the beginning, viewed as a voluntary commitment, since there was no intent to require practitioners already in service to become certified; Jordan notes that this approach is viable because "Death will eventually remove our individual deficiencies from the professional program."[13] Indeed! Training and certification certainly were needed; one growth area in particular was in the libraries being established in the hospitals of the U.S. Veterans Administration. To meet the needs of these VA hospitals, in a number of universities concentrated three-week courses began to be offered at library schools across the country, and these received the approval of the Medical Library Association. The number of practicing medical librarians had grown, and there was a need for meetings closer to home. Reports of various regional groups began to appear in the proceedings of the business meetings of the association.

From the beginning of training programs, North American medical librarians felt a responsibility to reach out internationally. The Rockefeller Foundation was persuaded to support fellowships for foreign medical librarians, and librarians from Chile, Cuba, Brazil, Uruguay, Ireland, Austria, and India were hosted as Rockefeller interns at American medical libraries. This international initiative was grounded in the idealism of the postwar period, and in the belief in a common purpose. It survives to the present through a legacy provided by Eileen R. Cunningham and the international outreach of North American medical librarians.

The medical library that was emerging in the postwar period required a new kind of librarian, and Mary Louise Marshall, president of the Medical Library Association, addressed the training needs for medical libraries during her presidency, careful to distinguish medical librarianship from general librarianship.[14] She speculated on the need for the establishment of standards of practice in medical librarianship. She recognized that the successful practice of modern librarianship will be based on the mastering of techniques, but, at the same time, that the librarian must be more than a master of processes: "The mastery of skills, techniques and routines should not be permitted to eclipse the many other characteristics which in sum characterize the successful librarian."[15] The concerns in 1946, when Marshall looked at the issue of education for medical librarianship, continued to require the attention of practicing medical librarians. Most medical librarians were entering professional practice with basic library training only. They acquired a familiarity with medical librarianship "on the job." In 1947 Columbia University School of Library Service began to address the special education of medical librarians through offering short courses in medical reference work, bibliography, administration, and hospital librarianship, which were attended by practicing medical librarians from the United States and Canada. To respond to this need, medical librarians adopted a training program at the annual meeting of the Medical Library Association in 1948, and a Code for the Training and Certification of Medical Libraries in 1949.

The preparation of a workforce of qualified and committed medical librarians continued to focus the energy of practicing medical librarians throughout the immediate postwar years. Following Mildred Jordan's spirited defense of certification, Janet Doe turned to the issue of education for medical librarianship in her presidential address.[16] She situates education for medical librarianship within the library school curriculum, as a medical course within the general curriculum, and argues for medical library internships as a means for acquiring subject knowledge. Janet Doe concluded her presidential address by reminding her audience of the views of Sir William Osler on library education, contained in his address at the opening of the Summer School of Library Service, Aberystwyth, Wales, in 1917. She refers to Osler's in-depth knowledge of the working procedures of libraries, and his concern for the lack of preparation for working in libraries. She concludes her presidential address with Osler's advice to librarians from his 1917 address: "Strive for mental accuracy and independence, cultivate the critical investigating faculty, keeping at the same time your mouth shut. In a profession demanding an amazing measure of equanimity, you cannot afford either to fight or to fret."[17] The spirit of Osler was very much with her!

The concern of education for medical librarianship was fully shared by Estelle Brodman. Marshall and Brodman worked closely together during this period on this critically important issue. Marshall referred in 1946 to Brodman's ideas on medical library education, although her article on this topic appeared only in the July 1949 issue of the *Bulletin of the Medical Library Association*. As the decade of the war ended, the leadership in the profession published a series of articles on education for medical librarianship.[18] Brodman, assistant librarian at Columbia University Medical Library, had been invited to speak at the annual meeting of the Medical Library Association about the work in education being done at the Columbia School of Library Service. Her paper sets forth the values and concepts of the program and provides a philosophy of education for the profession. She believed that students needed to be educated to rise to leadership positions in libraries. Educating students only in the techniques required for a first position cannot, Brodman argued, begin to justify the costs of postgraduate study in medical librarianship. Brodman describes the general Columbia program and discusses in detail the course in medical librarianship inaugurated by Thomas Fleming and subsequently taught by Brodman. This course was given in the spring semester, mainly to full-time students, and again in the summer, largely to permit practicing medical librarians to enroll. It consisted of two sections: medical literature and medical library administration. The improvement of education for medical librarianship was an essential initiative, one that needed to grow at schools across North America to satisfy the need that was to emerge in the 1950s for qualified medical librarians. Perhaps a personal anecdote may be permitted. As a newly graduated librarian from the University of Toronto's Graduate School in Library Science, I immigrated to the United States in 1962 and was offered the position of medical cataloger at the Lane Medical Library of Stanford University *before leaving Canada*. Librarians had remained in scarce supply as the expansion of the 1950s advanced. Doubtless, I would have greatly benefited from Brodman's course at Columbia, but the need for medical librarians was so great at the time that even a raw, foreign recruit, lacking any formal training in medical librarianship, could fill a need in a major medical library.

The decade that began with the threat of annihilation of all humanistic values was ending with a forceful commitment by medical librarians to excellence in performance standards and fundamental values. Making medical information available worldwide had a new and visible prominence. The cultural heritage issues raised when libraries were being destroyed had led to a determination to preserve the accumulated wisdom represented by the library. In her presidential address to the Medical Library Association in 1948, Eileen R. Cunningham speculated on the next fifty years of the work of medical librarians.[19] She had already made an enormous contribution through her work in containing the cost of foreign medical publications in the 1930s and her international outreach. She recognized the growth of the association with more medical, hospital, and dental librarians; more foreign members; and the need for collaboration with other associations. The first edition of the *Handbook of Medical Library Practice* had been published earlier in 1943 under the editorship of Janet Doe, and it was important that the success of this work in the service of improving the profession's standards of practice continue. Most significantly, Cunningham affirms the association as international in its mission. In a world where distances were shrinking, she comments:

> Our Association has always been a very internationally-minded group. Years ago we discussed the idea of adding the word "American" to our name. We decided against it because membership was not, then, and is not now, limited to any one country. Through the inauguration of our Committee on International and National Cooperation, we have been able to make our contacts and work more specific, and, we hope, more helpful in the international field. . . . There is, I believe, no more rewarding exercise in the world than the handclap of friendship extended over intervening miles and frontiers.[20]

INTO THE 1950s

Medical librarianship in the early 1950s was characterized by renewal of international ties and a time of optimism in the strengthening of international cooperation amongst medical libraries worldwide. For the first time medical librarians were to come together internationally at a congress. For several years, medical librarians worked diligently to prepare the program for the First International Congress on Medical Librarianship held in London, in July 1953, under the patronage of Sir Cecil Wakeley, president of the

Royal College of Surgeons of England. The continuation of these congresses to the present has played a major role in reenforcing core values. International cooperation could act as a deterrent to further conflagration and was on many agendas. The First World Conference on Medical Education was also held in London in 1953. Under the Medical Library Association's Committee on International Cooperation, medical librarians from countries such as Japan, India, and Argentina were visiting American libraries. UNESCO and the World Health Organization shared the vision of international medical library cooperation and provided support for study, travel, and training of librarians.

Nothing captures the contradictions of this era—the heightened idealism on the one hand and the growing threat of the Cold War and all its resulting paranoia on the other—so well as two short news items that appeared in 1953 in the pages of the *Bulletin of the Medical Library Association*. By January 1953, attendees from more than twenty countries had registered for the First International Congress on Medical Librarianship. The congress was to discuss the priority issues of training of medical librarians, the development and services of new medical libraries, and international cooperation among medical librarians.[21] The open, positive intent of the planners of this initiative can be seen in the program and attendance at this inaugural international congress on medical librarianship. Contrast this news item, if you will, with an unsigned editorial published a few months later.[22] Beginning with a general statement on the negative impact of war on libraries throughout history, the author comments, "The closed book and the closed mind are cause and effect; book burning by bigots and by fire bombers being the same results." One recalls the devastation of the Nazi bombings on the London libraries described in the *Bulletin* only a few years earlier. The anonymous author continues, noting that until recently, the impact of war on North American medical libraries had been largely on the budget due to wartime inflation, the lack of suitable staff due to drafting into the military, and the reduction of material due to printing priorities. But a different, more insidious threat to the library was beginning, one aimed at the role of the library as a transmitter of information, and one that struck directly at the core value of the profession, the provision of access to information. The author notes that many medical papers by military personnel were being published as "separates" in security classified documents, and therefore unavailable to a reader who has not received security clearance. The situation grew worse, apparently, due to the fact that mere security clearance was insufficient for access to these papers. The potential reader was required to demonstrate a reason for requiring access before reading the desired document. In a pessimistic conclusion, the editorial writer cautions that "the conflict between control of thought necessary for self-preservation in this time of real danger and our traditional freedom of thought vital to progress in science should be studied with great care and thoroughness." This tension was not new, and indeed is again evident in a post-9/11 world as librarians strive to keep their doors open and their resources accessible. Providing access to information, as a core professional value, has always required vigilance and courage on the part of librarians.

Prior to the outbreak of war, American medical librarians had been beset by problems in the delivery of medical information at the national level. War and recovery had delayed activities, but the time to return to this major issue had now arrived. The importance of a National Medical Library for medical librarians as well as physicians and researchers was clearly evident. Despite the energy and creativity of Billings, many of the problems had not been solved and the situation had deteriorated and was approaching crisis proportions, especially regarding the physical space and bibliographic control of the medical literature. Planning was complicated by old legislation that did not give a clear mandate to the Army Medical Library, as the National Library of Medicine was known at the time. It would seem that it was the fortitude and enthusiasm of Billings that had carved out a national role for the library. It also explains the difficulties in funding that had plagued this library at every innovative turn. Yet it was the only library in the United States fulfilling this role. The majority of the clients of the library were now civilians and the services were being provided by a military unit of the U.S. government. It was clear that new legislation was required to legitimize the de facto status of the National Medical Library and that the responsibility for the library needed, quite possibly, to be transferred to another agency of the government. The transfer to the Department of Health, Education and Security or annexation by the Library of Congress were only two of the scenarios being considered. These issues needed to be resolved before the necessary funding for the new building could be sought. Medical librarians were anxious for news of these developments, and Michael De Bakey, who was to play a long and distinguished role in the development of the library, was invited to update librarians on developments at an annual meeting in 1950. In doing so, De Bakey provided the library and medical librarians with a strong confirmation of their highest priority.

> I have come to believe that the primary function of a National Library
> of Medicine and its most important contribution to the advancement of

medical science is concerned with bibliographic control of current medical literature by means of special indexes and compilations. . . . A prompt comprehensive index to the current medical literature is of growing importance in this day of rapidly advancing scientific investigations.[23]

The need for adequate bibliographic control of the medical literature had national and international implications. Medical librarians were also assisted in their work by the International Federation for Documentation (FID) and the United Nations Educational, Scientific and Cultural Organizational (UNESCO). In 1949 UNESCO had intervened to maintain the nonprofit editorial work of Excerpta Medica. Excerpta Medica, an international specialty abstracting service covering both research and clinical findings, first appeared in 1947. This work helped medical librarians, especially in the print era, in bibliographic research which, as pointed out by De Bakey, was at the heart of their professional duties. A point of particular interest was the arrangements between Excerpta Medica and the Library of the Royal Netherlands Academy of Sciences to make microfiche copies of the abstracts of journals available to the subscribers of Excerpta Medica. Wilma Troxel was convinced that the intervention of UNESCO on the nonprofit issue resulted in a publication and a pricing system that was of greater benefit to medical librarians.[24] The nonprofit nature of the editorial function continued until 1971 when Excerpta Medica was acquired by the Elsevier Publishing Company; it represents one of the early mergers that by the 1990s were to be scrutinized and criticized by many medical librarians.

By the mid-1950s the medical community was focusing on machine methods as a means of improving access to medical information. The situation was increasingly urgent as research funding under "Big Science" initiatives was producing vast increases in the medical and scientific literature.[25] The Army Medical Library and the Welch Medical Library, Johns Hopkins University, had undertaken a major study to review the coverage of medical periodicals in the major abstracting and indexing services, employing IBM punched cards in conducting the study. It had been reported to Frank Rogers, director of the Army Medical Library, and his colleagues that the current way of managing access to medical literature was no longer viable. The groundwork was being laid for improved control of the medical literature that would make medical information indexing and dissemination a model in the library community. And by 1956, the enabling legislation that would make these developments possible was passed when

President Eisenhower signed Public Law 941 of the 84th Congress: *An Act to Establish a National Library of Medicine*. This legislation made it clear that the newly created National Library of Medicine was to act in the public good. By law, it held responsibility for medical information service to the medical profession and, through it, to the people of the United States.

A number of medical librarians had testified before Congress at the hearings regarding the development of a National Library of Medicine. Since the founding of the Medical Library Association, the Association's work had been shaped and facilitated by the work of the national library. The testimony of practicing librarians before the Congress on behalf of the National Medical Library was useful. It was also an acknowledgment of the integral relationship between medical librarians and the national library. Janet Doe, librarian of the New York Academy of Medicine, a past president of the Medical Library Association, and editor of two editions of the *Handbook of Medical Library Practice*, spoke strongly regarding the preeminent role of the library in providing access to the medical literature and of the rich and extensive collections housed in that library. Speaking on behalf of the medical library user who could not possibly afford to acquire all the books and journals needed in a personal library, she noted the reliance of the medical practitioner upon some four hundred medical libraries in the United States and Canada. At the time, three-quarters of these libraries had fewer than twenty thousand volumes, and 60 percent less than ten thousand. Clearly such collections could not be more than "working collections," and the more comprehensive collection at the national level which housed some six hundred thousand volumes at the time was essential. She addresses the authority to which the new national library should be responsible in clear and direct language.

> Now, why is it desirable to place this Library under another authority than the one which has built it to its present position? For a very specific reason. Its growth and efficiency while in the Army's hands vacillated distressingly between feast and famine. The 1944 Survey, made at the request of its enlightened and disturbed Director, described conditions of flagrant neglect, primarily due to the lack of continuity in direction inevitable under a change of head every four years. Its staff, untrained in librarianship, was pitifully few. Funds for books varied from year to year . . . in one two year period only sixteen books were bought.[26]

Having tackled this difficult political issue, Doe attacks with equal strength the need for a new library building:

But by far the most disheartening occurrence has been the absence of action by the Library's authorities towards securing new quarters for it. In 1944, the Survey wrote in capital letters as its first recommendation: "A NEW BUILDING IS AN ABSOLUTE NECESSITY." Twelve years have passed; efforts have been made repeatedly by the Library's staff to secure action. Last year the Library managed to get $350,000 included in the Navy's budget for building plans—and the money has failed to be used. This magnificent collection, unequalled anywhere in the world, is housed in an 1887 structure, non-fireproof, leaking in roof and windows, with stacks buckling and jammed with literature of incalculable value.[27]

The vigor of Janet Doe's testimony resounds to the present. Her passion for the cause leaps from the pages published a half century ago. The message is clearly contemporary as librarians for decades were to provide testimony to governments on behalf of the effective delivery of medical information in the public good.

By June 12, 1959, Senator Lister Hill shoveled the first earth at a ground breaking ceremony in Bethesda, Maryland, on the site of the new National Library of Medicine.[28] That same year, production of the *Index Medicus* began using the new mechanized system, with the first issue appearing in January 1960. The library had begun a massive, long-range overhaul of its indexing operations. Information technology would provide new, more efficient, timely, and comprehensive methods for the control of the literature. One of the basic indexing principles employed was that of a unit citation entry with a full citation appearing in all entries for a particular item. The automated unit entry could be recycled many times and appear in a variety of printed products. This concept of the single bibliographic entry was a key feature that reappeared later in the pioneer prototype of the integrated library system (ILS) developed in the 1970s by the library.

NOTES

1. Harold W. Jones, "The Role of Our National Medical Library in the Coming Era," *Bulletin of the Medical Library Association* 32, no. 4 (October 1944): 411.

The title of this editorial by the director of the Army Medical Library is of particular interest as he refers to the National Medical Library and not the actual title at the time, the Army Medical Library. This is recognition of the de facto role already played by the library and recognized by librarians for some time. Jones emphasizes this point when he states that he takes it for granted that librarians will recognize the reference to the Army Medical Library in his title.

2. Mary Louise Marshall, "The Library and Medical Education in Postwar Years" [editorial], *Bulletin of the Medical Library Association* 32, no. 4 (October 1944): 407–10.

3. L. T. Morton, "Foreign News" [letter], *Bulletin of the Medical Library Association* 30, no. 3 (April 1942): 226.

4. Victor Segalov, "Destruction of Russian Libraries," *A.L.A. Bulletin* 38 (1944): 215.

5. Eileen Cunningham and L. Marguerite Prime, "Expansion of the Cunningham Classification for Medical Literature," section on Military Medicine, XI–XII *Bulletin of the Medical Library Association* 31, no. 1 (January 1943): 67–75.

6. "Bibliography of War Medicine," *Bulletin of the Medical Library Association* 31, no. 1 (January 1943): 92–96.

7. "Foreign News," *Bulletin of the Medical Library Association* 30, no. 5 (October 1942): 476.

8. "Foreign News," *Bulletin of the Medical Library Association* 31, no. 2 (April 1943): 153.

9. "The American Book Center for War Devastated Libraries, Inc.," *Bulletin of the Medical Library Association* 33, no. 4 (October 1945): 532.

10. Ethel Wigmore, "The War and British Medical Libraries," *Bulletin of the Medical Library Association* 34, no. 3 (July 1946): 151–66.

11. Wigmore, "The War and British Medical Libraries," 160.

12. Mildred Jordan, "Certification: A Stage of Professionalism," *Bulletin of the Medical Library Association* 36, no. 2 (April 1948): 108–16.

13. Mildred Jordan, "Certification: A Stage of Professionalism," 116.

14. Mary Louise Marshall, "Training for Medical Librarianship," *Bulletin of the Medical Library Association* 34, no. 4 (October 1946): 247–52.

15. Leon Carnovsky, "Preparation for the Librarian's Profession," *Library Quarterly* 12 (1942): 404–11. Quoted by Marshall, p. 249.

16. Janet Doe, "The Development of Education for Medical Librarianship," *Bulletin of the Medical Library Association* 37, no. 3 (July 1949): 213–20.

17. Doe, "The Development of Education for Medical Librarianship," 220.

18. Doe, "The Development of Education for Medical Librarianship."

19. Eileen Cunningham, "The Association Faces the Next Fifty Years," *Bulletin of the Medical Library Association* 36, no. 4 (October 1948): 242–47.

20. Cunningham, "The Association Faces the Next Fifty Years," 246.

21. "News Items: The First International Congress on Medical Librarianship," *Bulletin of the Medical Library Association* 41, no. 1 (January 1953): 82.

22. "The Impact of Wars on Medical Libraries" [unsigned editorial], *Bulletin of the Medical Library Association* 41, no. 3 (July 1953): 290–91.

23. Michael E. De Bakey, "The Future of the Army Medical Library," *Bulletin of the Medical Library Association* 39, no. 2 (April 1951): 126.

24. Wilma Troxel, "International Medical Documentation: Present Status and Future Prospects," *Bulletin of the Medical Library Association* 40, no. 3 (July 1952): 278.

25. Derek J. de Solla Price, *Little Science, Big Science* (New York: Columbia University Press, 1963).

26. "A National Library of Medicine," Statement of Representative of Association of Senate Hearings, U.S. Congress, April 10, 1956, *Bulletin of the Medical Library Association* 44, no. 3 (July 1956): 371.

27. "A National Library of Medicine," 372.

28. Wyndham D. Miles, *A History of the National Library of Medicine, the Nation's Treasure of Medical Knowledge* (NIH Publication No. 82-1904) (Washington, DC: Government Printing Office, 1982), 484.

5

GAINING GROUND IN MEDICAL
LIBRARIES, 1960–1990

The activities that were undertaken to win the war and rebuild in the postwar decades created intellectual intensity and an investigative mentality that found new outlets in research. Medical research was transformed by the availability of large-scale funding. The "war" metaphor was sustained as researchers now were ready to make war, not on human beings, but on the diseases of human beings. The power of medical research that had been directed to war medicine—infection, trauma, emergency surgery, tropical disease, venereal disease, as priorities—was now ready to serve the diseases of a civilian population—cancer, cardiovascular disease, arthritis. Scott Adams has admirably captured this period of intensive, well-funded and highly focused medical research and its impact on medical information and bibliography.[1] During this period, the complex relationships between governments, universities, and the private sector that is the basis of research were shaped. In the process, medicine was becoming more interdisciplinary and more technologically dependent. These developments altered medical libraries as well, challenging medical librarians to revise their methods of delivery of medical information. They also laid the groundwork for even greater and more formalized library cooperation at the regional, national, and international levels. The efforts of medical librarians in the United States to meet these new challenges were facilitated by two major developments: a new National Library of Medicine and the Medical Library Assistance Act of 1965. As the National Library of Medicine explored the use of advanced information technology to improve the communication of medical research results, it was to provide medical librarians around the world with powerful new tools for the delivery of medical information.

The economy of North America in the 1960s was enjoying a period of growth and confidence. New medical schools were being established, and those already in existence were paying attention to the importance of the library and its role in medical education. Standards of practice and performance for medical librarians were being confirmed through certification and teaching programs that had begun a decade earlier. For the first time at its annual meeting in 1961, the Medical Library Association offered an advanced seminar in searching the medical literature open to medical librarians who worked with collections of more than ten thousand volumes. At the same time, the importance of using the emerging information technologies to improve access to medical literature was growing. Subject control of a large and highly specialized knowledge base was a fundamental issue. The use of IBM punched cards, sorting machines, and coordinate indexing characterized this period. In its simplest form, coordinate indexing represented the combining of simple, elementary terms. In the increasingly interdisciplinary literature of biomedicine, the combined term searches were essential for medical librarians to gain better access to the literature. The use of punched cards and combined keyword searching gave promise of new machine methods for controlling the medical literature and making it available. Medical librarians throughout North America were faced with difficult choices as well in the organization of their libraries. The work completed a decade earlier on the classification of medical library collections by the National Library of Medicine[2] required that medical librarians review whatever system they presently were using, and make the decision of whether the large effort of reclassification of a book collection was justified by the resulting improvement in control of the literature.

Work was also under way for a second International Congress on Medical Librarianship to be held in Washington, D.C., a full ten years after the inaugural conference in London. The U.S. National Library of Medicine was to make an exceedingly important contribution to this meeting, as Frank Rogers, director of the National Library of Medicine, was chairman of the congress. The congress theme, "Libraries in the Advancement of Medicine," gave ample opportunity to the medical library community to demonstrate their core professional mission of providing access to medical information. Papers were needed on topics that represented the major issues in the practice of medical librarianship during this period: library organization, especially in libraries in the undeveloped areas; library resources; training and education for medical librarianship; medical library history; and a growing area of mechanization and automation in libraries.

A new method for producing the *Index Medicus*, by now a standard tool worldwide for medical librarians, had been created. Progress depended upon the intense collaboration of the Council on Library Resources, the

Institute for Scientific Information, and the remarkable talent of Eugene Garfield, who had participated in the earlier Welch Medical Library Indexing Project. Under the leadership of the National Library of Medicine, Frank B. Rogers and Seymour I. Taine transformed the *Index Medicus*. From today's digital perspective, it is difficult to imagine that when this work was done, the problem of appropriate photographic equipment was a key concern in the improvement of the production of the Index. Eastman Kodak's Listomatic camera was chosen by the National Library of Medicine. Composition of text, punched card preparation, and all related operation costs were all components in the major redesign of a system. The objective was increased coverage, accuracy, and timeliness of content. The efforts that led to these improvements were well documented in the pages of the *Bulletin of the Medical Library Association*.[3]

The transformation that the Index was undergoing gave medical librarians working in all libraries essential improvements in the provision of access to medical information. It marked the beginning of the application of increasingly sophisticated technological methods to the control of the medical literature. Such a major revision of a tool that medical librarians around the world used on a daily basis was certainly the subject of much discussion among medical librarians. Although North Americans had more opportunities to learn and discuss these developments as the project evolved, discussion was not limited to that continent. In his regular "Notes from London," Leslie Morton reports on lively discussion within the Medical Section of the Library Association. Discussion here reflected an international issue—the use of English translations of foreign titles in the new version.[4] Leslie Morton's short summary of this discussion concludes with the hope that these comments will not be interpreted ungraciously, as there was great gratitude to the United States for the production of the *Index Medicus*.

The complete integration of the products and services of the National Library of Medicine into the work of medical librarians, nationally and internationally, was evident. There remained the matter of a new building for the National Library of Medicine, which was reported to medical librarians in an issue of the *Bulletin of the Medical Library Association*[5] under the guest editorship of the director of the National Library of Medicine. The National Library and the Medical Library Association saw their roles as reaching out to other nations and librarians, recognizing that full control of the medical literature worldwide required partnership in recording the literature. They worked to provide access to the medical literature through identifying national medical indexes and in so doing laid the groundwork for an international network of medical libraries.

These federally funded initiatives in the United States were not characteristic of other nations. But in Canada, many of the same economic, scholarly, and technological influences were at work. The first effort to provide a comprehensive, quantitative survey of libraries serving medical schools in Canada appeared in 1964.[6] The Association of Canadian Medical Colleges provided initiative and support for this landmark study, the stimulation for which began during discussions at a Canadian Medical School Group dinner held during the 1959 annual meeting of the Medical Library Association in Toronto. Beatrice Simon's study described the collections, services, and support of the eleven medical school libraries that existed at that time in Canada. Simon's report provided recommendations for Canada, including a national coordinated medical information service that would have responsibility for the MEDLARS[7] program in Canada and a national medical bibliographic center. On the whole the recommendations of Simon's report were to be implemented, but not always in the manner she had envisioned. One recommendation, regarding cooperative collection development in Canadian medical libraries, retains historical interest as an unmet challenge to collaboration:

> Retrospective collections of foreign language publications could also be developed on a cooperative basis. Toronto already leads in coverage of the journals published in Great Britain and Ireland; Laval has a large number of French language periodicals and receives currently more medical publications from French speaking countries than any other library; McGill's holdings of German and Swiss publications are extensive and need not be duplicated elsewhere except as local libraries might wish to have outstanding current titles. British Columbia and McGill happen to be rivals in collecting Russian, Scandinavian and Swiss periodicals, but need both libraries build up huge back files of these?[8]

Implicit in this challenge is the recognition that at the time of Simon's report there was no support at the national level for a strong collection of medical documents to support the national infrastructure of medical libraries. Simon's intellectual challenge thrown to the academic medical librarian community was not met, as Simon anticipated, by the creative collaboration of medical librarians. Rather, restructuring resulted from the combination of an increasingly unilingual English-speaking medical community (except in French Canada) and budget reductions that forced journal cancellations of less-used materials, many of them in languages other than English. Nonetheless, Simon's *Library Support of Medical Education and*

Research in Canada was a foundation document by one of Canada's most influential medical librarians. As both a medical librarian and a university librarian, Beatrice Simon made major contributions to the improvement of libraries and information delivery in Canada.

In Canada, there was a growing need to formalize the relationship between academic medical libraries that resulted in the establishment in 1967 of a Standing Committee on Medical School Libraries of the Association of Canadian Medical Colleges/L'Association des facultés de médecine du Canada. Canadian medical school librarians had been brought together through their attendance at annual meetings of the Medical Library Association, but the opportunity to meet as a uniquely Canadian group was provided by the creation of this new committee. The same year, 1967, the National Science Library of Canada had been mandated as the center for coordinated support to medical libraries through the creation of a Health Sciences Resource Centre for Canada within the National Science Library.[9] This was to be the home of MEDLARS in Canada under the international outreach program of the National Library of Medicine. These two Canadian developments indicate an increasing need for librarians to develop nationally based institutions to serve the advancement of medical libraries. At the same time, while becoming national, the core value of access to medical information was being reenforced.

THE 1970s

Advances in information technology, the growth of the medical and scientific literature, and the strong leadership and collaboration of the National Library of Medicine and the medical library community made possible the dynamic changes of the 1970s. The mandate of the National Library of Medicine had been clarified and broadened and the Medical Library Assistance Act of 1965 (MLAA) passed a decade earlier. This had laid the groundwork for addressing the challenge faced by U.S. medical libraries in addressing the imbalance between library resources and the information needs of library users. The MLAA provided libraries with much needed funding and, more important, developed a regional medical library network linking the National Library of Medicine with regional medical libraries across the country. This network of medical libraries provided an organizational model to medical libraries in other countries and suggested a leadership role for national libraries in ensuring access to medical information that continues to the present.

During the first five years of the MLAA (1965–1970), the medical library community in the United States witnessed the addition of more than forty-three million dollars under a system of grants and contracts designed to correct the imbalance between physicians' needs and the librarians' resources. Improving libraries through grants required reliable statistical information, including directories of medical libraries and collection statistics on the libraries. Information on growth in the numbers of health professionals was needed better to estimate the increased demands that were being placed upon the services and collections of medical libraries. In early efforts to compile sound statistics on medical libraries in the United States, Alan Rees noted in an article written in 1972 that in 1960 there were 86 medical schools in the United States, and by 1969, 103 schools existed.[10] A library was required for a medical school to be accredited, and the quality of the services and collections was a concern, since librarians had to acquire and make available medical information that was growing at an exponential rate. They also needed to use new methods of information management if they were to provide the necessary services. By the 1970s, eleven medical school libraries had been designated under the National Library of Medicine's Regional Medical program,[11] and MEDLARS search centers had been set up in many others. A statistical snapshot of medical school libraries, hospital libraries, libraries serving the allied health professions, and society libraries was prepared under a grant from the National Library of Medicine, documenting the challenges for the decade ahead.[12] The MLAA provided financing for core activities and for the construction of facilities. It also enabled training in medical librarianship, publishing in biomedicine, and the Regional Medical Library (RML) program.

Medical Library Leadership: Reflections on the 1970s

In a special issue of *Library Trends*,[13] leaders in American medical librarianship described state-of-the-art developments in the mid-1970s. Issue editor Joan Titley Adams chose well in selecting her contributors, whose influence on medical library developments extended from the end of World War II until the 1980s. The changes medical librarianship had undergone in recent decades, present projects, and future trends were all captured in this extraordinary set of articles. Many of these developments in medical libraries were the direct result of the enormous changes in health care and the medical profession, new and accelerated production of knowledge, and changes in the education of health professionals. These changes propelled medical librarianship forward, encouraging medical librarians to advance bibliographic control of the biomedical literature and to promote access to documents, and they helped to reinforce the core value of librarians in providing access to medical information. As already mentioned, by the mid-1970s, the Medical Library Assistance Act had been in place for a decade, the MEDLARS program was mature, and the Regional Medical Library program was fully functional. These developments significantly altered medical libraries, and one, the MEDLARS program, was to have international significance. Advanced bibliographic access, automated indexing and online searching were fully available although only within the walls of the library. Access to health information had improved enormously through interlibrary cooperation and the organized lending under the Regional Medical Library Program of the U.S. National Library of Medicine. New medical libraries were being built and existing ones renovated under the funding provided by NLM grants. And education for medical librarianship was being reviewed. These improvements were creating a revitalization of medical librarianship and reinforcing core professional values, especially in the area of access to medical information. The result was a dynamic period in the profession of medical librarianship. Looking backward to the 1960s, Mildred Langner in her contribution to this special issue reflects on developments as follows:

> Throughout all the turbulence, librarians attempted to give the scientific research worker the best possible service, but neither they, nor perhaps even the researcher himself, knew exactly what was needed for the library.[14]

Science and medicine had grown in scale and complexity and were making demands that could be met only by a more sophisticated library using new management techniques and state-of-the-art information technology. Langner's observation was no longer correct, as medical librarians, especially those in leadership roles, had to know where the library needed to go and be able to take it there. The demand by medical librarians for continuing education programs in medical library management and planning during the 1970s verified this trend. Medical librarians worked to upgrade their knowledge and skills in this dynamic and demanding environment. Many had not received specialized professional training, as noted elsewhere. Nonetheless, they were providing advanced specialized services in their libraries, largely as the result of on-the-job learning, training programs, and continuing education courses, offered by the Medical Library Association and many database providers who understood that training needed to be part of their marketing efforts.

In the same issue of *Library Trends*, Louise Darling describes the changes in medical librarianship in the 1970s, and in doing so, articulates a core value of the profession: "Health sciences librarians are likely to identify closely with users of their libraries because of the human and humanitarian appeal of the subject area."[15]

A sense of identity with the community served continues to characterize medical library practice. Darling also identifies concerns that were becoming evident in the inequality in levels of service available, most especially in nonteaching hospitals. Much had been done to improve access and outreach under the Regional Medical Library program, but it was becoming clear that much remained to be done. Darling further notes that equalization of access to medical information is a continuing preoccupation of medical librarians, much to their credit. Darling's own work as biomedical librarian, University of California, Los Angeles, and director of the Pacific Southwest Regional Medical Library Service demonstrated this determination to provide access to heath information to all who need to use it.

Online Bibliographic Access Comes of Age

In retrospect, the 1970s appear as a halcyon period in the advancement of access to medical information. Developments in the Internet era were still more than a decade ahead, but maximum use of information technology, as it was understood in the 1970s, was in place in many medical libraries in the developed world. One of the more prescient initiatives of this period was the development of the AIM-TWX service at a number of U.S. medical school libraries. This early experiment in online retrieval of the medical literature, using a database that consisted of the article citations in the *Abridged Index Medicus* (AIM) was an indication of the possibility of online searching that changed fundamentally the access to medical literature in the Internet era. AIM-TWX was a remote-access bibliographic control-and-retrieval system developed for the Lister Hill National Center for Biomedical Communications by the System Development Corporation. TWX was a teletype terminal. Searching of the AIM database used a controlled vocabulary, MeSH (Medical Subject Heading List of the National Library of Medicine). These early experiments revealed the need for intensive training programs if the online retrieval system was to be used effectively. The use of telecommunications to improve access to medical information was in its infancy, and there were many problems: the machine itself, the communication line between the machine and the host computer, and computer malfunctioning. Not the least of the tensions in these early experiments were the line charges and the costs of a search. But the potential of online, multiterm machine searching was clearly demonstrated by these early experiments, and the drive to provide a fully effective system was on.

Improved library operations using automation were encouraged under the MLAA. Several significant examples highlight both the importance of this grants program and the determination of librarians to improve their internal operations. Under the NLM grant, the UCLA Biomedical Library developed an online serials control system to support serials processing, references, check-in, claims, and binding—all activities that were under great pressure due to the increase in the amount of information libraries were processing.[16] These early improvements using information technology served as models and provided medical librarians, both in the United States and elsewhere, with proven solutions to real workplace needs. One of the most important product improvements of the period was in the production of union lists of serials using computer technology; these lists helped to encourage effective sharing of library holdings among peers, especially hospital librarians, to aid in the rationalization of collections. The University of Minnesota Biomedical Library received a National Library of Medicine Grant[17] in 1972 to develop a prototype computer-based library management system that would be both affordable and appropriate in medium-size and large medical libraries. The basic concept, today commonplace in all commercially available integrated library systems, was one integrated system for management of all medical library processing. Another feature of the work done in Minnesota was that both the equipment and the software would be developed as a package, thus freeing librarians from the high costs of development, allowing the equipment and software to be maintained by nontechnical people, and contractual arrangements. The 1970s was a heady time of development and experimentation with computers in medical libraries. Medical librarians made rapid progress in the discovery of technological solutions, aided and guided by the programs of the National Library of Medicine.

Librarians in both the developed and the developing world outside of the United States looked to U.S. libraries for solutions to their information-processing needs. In particular, they saw the development of MEDLARS as a major step and became active in their efforts to provide MEDLARS service within their countries. Acting on behalf of medical libraries in the developing world, the World Health Organization established a WHO MEDLINE Centre in Geneva in 1972, at first processing searches on MEDLARS tapes supported at the Biomedical Documentation Centre in Stockholm and in 1974 converting to online operations. In the first eighteen months, the

WHO MEDLINE Centre performed 4,079 searches, 65 percent of which were for member countries of WHO, the majority of which were countries in the developing world.[18] The challenges faced by libraries in the developing world in the use of MEDLARS were enormous. American MEDLARS was built upon a sound infrastructure of regional document delivery, librarian training programs, and library improvement grants. The developing world had no such infrastructure on which to build, and from the inception of the WHO initiative, the challenges were different from those in the developed world. Following the announcement of the availability of the service, the response of potential users was low, or the announcement misunderstood, a frequent misunderstanding being that MEDLINE was a document provider, not a literature-searching service. Perhaps this was wishful thinking on the part of some of the users who relied upon collections in their home libraries that were far from adequate. Training was a key issue in promoting the acceptance of MEDLINE in the developing world, and WHO began to invest in training programs for their member countries. Careful planning and promotion took place, enabling the libraries to begin to take advantage of MEDLARS on behalf of their users.

One of the major stumbling blocks for the developing world was the fundamental issue of the quality of collections at the local level and the need for improvement in document delivery. If a medical library facility existed at all, it was often far from adequate. The litany of problems faced by medical librarians would have daunted many of their colleagues from the developed world: inadequate collections, including many broken runs of journals; lack of staff training and retraining; lack of equipment; a very poorly developed philosophy of resource sharing and interlibrary cooperation. But these challenges presented the opportunity to begin to address the problems, and document delivery received assistance through free photocopy services supplied by the National Library of Medicine and the British Council. On a library-to-library basis, medical libraries in the developed world began to "twin" with developing world libraries to improve access to information, a process that continued for decades to follow. Estelle Brodman had anticipated many of these infrastructure barriers to the improvement of the delivery of medical information worldwide. She had visited many libraries in Europe, India, Thailand, Taiwan, and Japan, and spoke with her customary keenness and vigor on the issue of the need to improve collections, the quality of staff and the training of staff, library buildings, and telephone and electrical services. Brodman was not discussing MEDLARS; her concern was the overall condition of medical libraries worldwide. Her remarks make interesting reading today for their power to focus on what really matters in the provision of access to information. She issues a challenge to medical librarians worldwide to become less passive in their delivery of medical information, to demonstrate their competence, to study their communities, and to become a part of them. Above all she reminds us that the road to effective library services does not have a "magic bullet":

> The worse the librarian and the less capable of coping with the problems the library is, the more is he likely to think that computers will solve all his troubles—and that without his having to do any deep thinking or performing any hard work. This is true in poor, struggling libraries in the small hospitals in the Midwest United States; it is even truer of libraries in Indonesia, India and Nepal where the difficulty of getting another staff member or typewriter is as great as that of getting a computer. Such librarians, of course, have given up hope and are generally clutching at straws. And medical libraries seem particularly prone to it, perhaps as a result of the ease with which they can receive MEDLARS searches.[19]

Trouble in Paradise

Federal support under the MLAA created an expectation of continuity on behalf of many U.S. medical librarians. The growth and innovation that it made possible was viewed as essential, and therefore the renewal of this support by the U.S. Congress was viewed as equally essential. But times were changing, medical care delivery was changing, and library users were changing. The desire to expand health care to a larger segment of the American population through prepayment plans and government support was advancing. New areas of collections in medical libraries were developing in health care economics, the sociology of medicine, and public aspects of medicine. The oil crisis of the early 1970s showed cracks in the system. The economic crisis provoked by the oil embargo reduced government support in other areas such as biomedical research, which in turn impacted on libraries just at the time of critical experimentations in new techniques in medical information management and the growth of information that the library needed to acquire. Estelle Brodman cast a critical eye on the achievements under the Medical Library Assistance Act and looked for changes in concept in the extension of the Act, noting that less had been done for medical libraries than had originally been hoped. She summarized the situation for medical libraries:

> Libraries are like the disadvantaged in our culture, the last to be given extensive funding through grants and subventions and the first to lose

these when the economic situation becomes tight. Libraries, therefore, like the poor, never have the feeling of certainty and assurance of continued funding that is part of the background of some other parts of our economy. As Scott Adams once noted, libraries are so unused to having money that they don't know how to use it when they have it.[20]

Other clouds were on the horizon. It was not until 1975 that the bitterly contested claim against NLM by the publisher Williams & Wilkins was finally resolved. As technology advanced, it had improved the ability of libraries to share resources through providing photocopies of needed material. Beginning with the rebuilding of service after the end of Word War II, the amount of photocopy provided by the National Library of Medicine had continued to increase. Beginning in 1957, the National Library of Medicine ceased to lend physical copies, providing photocopies of requested materials instead, and as the years went by, publishers expressed concern over revenue loss resulting from extensive photocopying. By 1968, William N. Passano, president of Williams & Wilkins, was expressing the concerns of that firm regarding photocopying at the National Library of Medicine, and asked that a royalty of two cents per page be paid. The NLM director, Martin Cummings, invoked the "fair use" exemption, a sort of informal agreement under copyright allowing the NLM to make single copies for individual use by scholars. Failing to achieve its commercial objective of two cents per page per copy, on February 27, 1968, Williams & Wilkins filed a petition against the government, alleging that the National Library of Medicine had infringed the copyright of materials.[21] This suit had serious implications for the National Library of Medicine and for other medical libraries. It was an early and serious skirmish in the beginning of the "Copyright Wars" that continue to the present and are discussed in chapter 12, on copyright. The case for the National Library of Medicine was built on the argument that all research resulting from public funding and described in a document held by the library could be freely copied. This argument has persisted to the present, although it should be noted that the stronger case was made on the doctrine of "fair use."

After a see-saw battle, the Court of Claims finally ruled by one vote, that the making of single copies of journal articles did not violate existing law. This decision was appealed to the U.S. Supreme Court by Williams & Wilkins, and in 1975, the decision of the Court of Claims was upheld. This important victory, reaffirming the right of public institutions to provide access to information, was truly precedent-setting. Miles claims in his institutional history of the National Library of Medicine that for Martin Cummings, the director of the National Library of Medicine, "it was the most trying event during his term as Director. For years he devoted half of his time to the case. It sapped more of his energy than all other problems combined, and he felt that it triggered the heart attack that sent him to the hospital in 1973."[22] The timing of this decision had implications for the review of American copyright legislation that was underway. Less than two years later, new copyright replaced the legislation of 1909, and embedded in this new legislation was the vital principle of "fair use" that limited the exclusive rights of publishers and enthroned the ability of libraries to act responsibly but to continue to provide photocopies of journal articles for the public good. It was not until the digital era that this right was again in jeopardy.

Ethics, Values, and Medical Libraries: A View from the 1970s

As the decade of the 1970s drew to a close, Helen Crawford, a past president of the Medical Library Association (1972) and onetime director of the Middleton Health Sciences Library, University of Wisconsin, reflected on ethics and values in medical librarianship, a rare topic for the *Bulletin of the Medical Library Association*. Before turning to Crawford's comments, it is important to distinguish between professional ethics and values. Statements of professional ethics provide codes of conduct for members of a profession. Professional values help to define and inform codes of ethics, but are neither prescriptive not compulsory. Values help to determine career choice and professional behavior. Crawford's essential concern is ethics, but in the course of her discussion she sheds light upon fundamental values in medical librarianship. Crawford begins her discussion by recognizing the lack of documented concern for the ethic of medical librarianship. She finds evidence of this lacuna in the third edition of the *Handbook of Medical Library Practice*, which contains no reference to ethics in its index.

Her no-nonsense approach to this question prompts her to note that a large number of codes of ethics for libraries in general exist, but the necessary power to regulate and enforce these codes does not exist in many cases. Further, since by the late 1970s the number of these codes had proliferated, she questions the need for a code for medical librarians in particular. Her article is interesting in the contrast it demonstrates to today's world and the practice of medical librarianship. She says, for example, "Because of its specialized clientele and limited subject field, the medical library escapes some of the pressures on the public library—for instance, problems of censorship, conformance with local norms and commitment to serve all elements of society."[23]

A basic premise of this book is that medical libraries share a commitment to provide medical information to all who need to use it, a statement that Crawford's comments might appear to challenge. In part II of this book, we shall explore this commitment further, showing how communications technology has enhanced the ability of librarians to fulfill this commitment. Crawford's statement reminds us that providing service to a larger community was more restricted and less feasible in the pre-Internet era.

Another contrast between the 1970s and the present era is reflected in a further statement by Crawford: "How many of you have considered that medical libraries are in a monopoly position within their immediate communities. They have the technical materials and specialized staff and control access to the bibliographic apparatus of their discipline."[24] In today's world, the idea that a librarian occupies a privileged, indeed a monopolistic, position with respect to the provision of information is far from reality. While many of the developments and improvements in the delivery of medical information have been generated by a genuine desire to improve access to medical information for all who need to use it, much of the reengineering of the library has been the result of the pressures of a competitive market in the information age. Today it is no longer true that the librarian holds the key to the information kingdom, if she ever did. There are alternatives that can and do bypass the library, most especially those that are provided by the Internet.

And consider her further description of the medical librarian,

> The modern generation of MEDLARS searchers (the contemporary equivalent of Dean Wilson's vestal virgins guarding the portal of knowledge) may well do more for the image of the medical library than all our efforts in public relations. User and librarian share in this modern mystery through the face-to-face interview, the painstaking search of the maze, and the suspense of waiting for the oracle to respond. It is odd that a technical advance should have such a humanizing effect.[25]

How the world has changed! Few medical librarians today would look back longingly on playing the role of vestal virgin at the gates of knowledge, also known as librarian-mediated searching. The empowerment of the user through educational and training programs provided by the medical library has happily replaced the guardian of the gates of knowledge. But discussion of historic differences does not demean the value in much of what Crawford has to say. She encouraged thoughtful reflection on the part of the medical library community on why librarians do what they do. She also helps to set the stage for discussion on consumer health information and clinical information that intensifies over the next decades, as shown in her following comment,

> Medical librarians at all levels must come to grips with the issue of pa-
> tient education. Some years ago an article indicated that hospital staff in
> training was infinitely more comfortable when dealing with the physical
> ills of patients than when dealing with the social problems. Medical li-
> brarians are in this position with regard to patient education: Our hold-
> ings, our book selection habits, our reference tools, and our professional
> orientation are all geared toward support of scientific work. We are un-
> comfortable with patients and their relatives and with laymen in general,
> uneasy at intruding upon the doctor-patient relationship, and fearful of
> doing harm. Our hospital library colleagues are ahead of the rest of us
> in dealing constructively with the layman's need for medical information
> but they should not have to deal with it alone.[26]

Helen Crawford has given us a mature view of the issue of ethics, values, and commitment by the medical librarian during a decade that emphasized technology and managerial competencies in an increasingly expanding and sophisticated information environment. If values and ethics
became de-emphasized during this period, they would be restored in later
decades as the tools to broaden their services and expand their roles became
more available to the medical library community.

THE 1980s

The significant advancement of medical libraries in the 1970s provided the
basis for further developments in the 1980s. Although the model of the library was changing, the three core values of librarians—acting in the public good by providing access to health information for all who need to use
it, educating users in accessing information, and preserving the history of
medical and health science—had remained intact. One of the strongest factors that contributed to this survival was the ability of the medical librarian
to adapt to change. And the environment in which librarians practiced their
profession experienced accelerated change as the decade advanced. An increasing and costly investment in technology in all sectors of society, an emphasis on cost awareness and cost effectiveness, higher accountability with
regard to the use of public funds especially in the fields of education and
health care, and a demand on the part of the taxpayer for more and better
services—all of these factors had a role to play in the direction the medical

library took in the 1980s. Medical knowledge production was on an extended exponential growth curve, and publishing and information availability was on the way to becoming very big business if it had not already reached that point. Success in the library was determined by the degree to which the organization could adapt and provide improved services in this changing environment.

Despite past successes, and as we have seen, they were many, the medical library needed to be reconceptualized. The need for a visionary rethinking was filled by Nina Matheson and John A. Cooper in a highly influential report commissioned by the Association of American Medical Colleges and funded in part by the National Library of Medicine.[27] In their opinion, the inadequacies of American medical libraries had been addressed by the Medical Library Assistance Act and the leadership role of the U.S. National Library of Medicine. Physical facilities were improved and intellectual resources strengthened. By the early 1980s, according to Matheson and Cooper, few libraries were in need of physical replacement and collections were reasonably adequate. Online medical information, MEDLARS, and expert knowledge systems in, for example, human genetics, were being developed. The major challenge of the 1980s was the shift from a paper-based system in the delivery of medical information to a fully electronic medical information delivery system. Obvious as this reality is in our own day, the clear call to action to implement this paradigm shift was a wake-up call: "The societal view of the importance of individual access to and control of information is changing: in a highly competitive technologically based world, individuals and organizations with better quality information services are more productive and effective."[28]

A new role for the medical librarian was emerging in the application of appropriate new technologies to information and libraries. Librarians would be called upon to assist faculty and students in their development of skills in medical information access and information management. The key role of librarian as educator was gaining new prominence in the information age, and the core value of providing access to information through information literacy was being redefined and reinforced.

Another important need that Matheson and Cooper foresaw was the integration of information resources within the academic health sciences center, a need that could be filled by the librarian acting as the manager of all institutional information resources, not only those traditionally provided by the medical library. The "Matheson Report" as this report came to be called, emphasized the important role that the library could play as a change agent and its responsibility in advancing an integrated health information network. An approach that was both positive and proactive on the part of medical librarians was bound to find numerous advocates both in the U.S. medical librarian community and beyond. It challenged the stereotype of libraries by proposing that they could become change centers. Full library automation of all operations was a necessary first step. The U.S. National Library of Medicine was proposed as the change engine and the leadership provider for these major changes to the nation's medical libraries and their medical educational programs. The report's conclusion and recommendations were directed to all players involved in health care—the academic health sciences centers, professional associations, and public and private agencies. Almost a quarter century later, the "Matheson Report" continues to challenge, for it was one of the first documents in library and information management to address the needs of the information age in a comprehensive manner. In so doing, Matheson and Cooper also provided a new language for medical libraries in the information age.

Medical librarians had created many of the improvements on which this new vision of the integrated academic information resource would be founded. Nina Matheson, assistant director of Health Information Management Studies, Association of American Medical Colleges, capitalized on the collective wisdom of the medical library leadership in the United States and Canada in her Delphi Study of 1982.[29] Her methodology was well chosen and her perceptive analysis provided a study that still makes interesting reading. She shows us what the medical library leadership of the moment saw and failed to see in their environment:

> The data suggest that the library directors perceive the adoption of technology as desirable and within the libraries' decision span. Education and service roles of librarians will expand. Technology is most desired when it enhances present practices, and where the library as an autonomous, central information source is continued. Library and institutional priorities are perceived as obstacles to change. Librarians appear to lack necessary motivation and skills to assume different roles. Directors seem to seek to extend present services to other user groups (consumers, public and patients) rather than develop new services for primary users. Respondents appear to be saying that change will occur, but there will always be libraries as we know them.[30]

Matheson's Delphi Study involved medical librarians ranking a set of statements on a scale of one to seven with respect to the desirability and probability of a given statement. It is interesting to revisit some of these statements and their ranking a quarter of a century later and to reflect upon what librarians then thought about the future of their profession. All statements and their ranking are taken directly from the published study. Medical library directors were asked to respond to a number of propositions, and their replies identify many tensions within medical librarianship:

"A gradual but positive shift to electronic forms of texts of books and journals will take place. Private industry will control access to these files and provide text on demand for fees."

Desirable: 11.3%

Probable: 30.0%

"Personal microcomputers and stand-alone information systems will make a rapid appearance in all health care and teaching settings. They will be linked to remote information sources and bypass libraries as traditional information sources."

Desirable: 13.5%

Probable: 26.3%

"With the advent of computer-based diagnostic information systems and knowledge data banks, the use of libraries by clinicians as sources of information will decline."

Desirable: 6.0%

Probable: 20.35%

"The library will assume the role of coordinator and manager of the academic health center's total information delivery efforts."

Desirable: 71.3%

Probable: 19.9%

"Users of knowledge and information data bases will need information resource consultants to teach them efficient methods of data base access."

Desirable: 85.7%

Probable: 77.0%

"Providing consumer health information and meeting needs of consumer's "right to knowledge" will become a regular function in health sciences libraries."

Desirable: 68.4%

Probable: 57.9%

"Through the electronic medium the library will transcend its physical boundaries by communicating directly with remote users and delivering information to them in their homes and work sites. The concept of the user always having to go to the library will disappear."

Desirable: 29.2%

Probable: 28.8%"

"Libraries will fail to initiate new educational and clinically based information delivery programs. Other agencies will fill the vacuum, leaving libraries with the traditional roles of managing study halls and storage bins."

Desirable: 0.8%

Probable: 5.3%

"Teaching methods of accessing computer-based information systems to health students will become a paramount role and primary responsibility of academic librarians."

Desirable: 41.7%

Probable: 27.1%

"Library schools and other knowledge-management faculties will gear admission requirements and educational programs to meet new demands."

Desirable: 93.7%

Probable: 13.7%

These specific statements and their evaluations have been quoted to show gaps between the desirable and the probable and the difficulties perceived by librarians at the time in achieving desired outcomes. It is clear that some librarians, in many cases the majority of the library leadership at the time in the United States and Canada who completed the Delphi survey, felt some developments desirable but not achievable. Some of the results reflect a collective misreading of the future by the participants, who were in some measure responsible for the creation of that future. If librarians in the survey were less than fully successful in predicting the future, they should not be chastised, since there is cloud in most crystal balls. They were, however, quite prophetic about the role of the library in the delivery of consumer health information and the necessary changes in the library profession.

The Delphi Study and the Matheson-Cooper report launched a rethinking of the medical library in the 1980s. What strikes a reader twenty-five years later is the reaffirmation of the core values of the profession that were transferred into an increasingly advanced technological environment. A firm commitment to service drives the desire, indeed, the enthusiasm to adapt the library, to change the shape of the medical library, but not the fundamental values that had defined the profession throughout its history. But the point of these studies was not the affirmation of core values but the identification of new roles for the medical librarian in a changing environment.

The response of medical librarians was not entirely uniform in the acceptance of this new role. An exchange of letters in the *Bulletin of the Medical Library Association* between David Bishop, university librarian, University of California, San Francisco, and Nina Matheson, then at the National Library of Medicine, serve to illustrate this point.[31]

Bishop's concern was with what he perceived as a single homogeneous model that might suit some but not necessarily all academic health centers and their libraries. Further, he saw this model as one that was derived from the industrial, corporate, or commercial world. A further concern was the readiness of the staff in many medical libraries to manage information of certain kinds. In his opinion, the management of clinical laboratory data or data for decision making in health care planning was outside the purview of the medical library. Matheson's response is that her research has suggested a new model for the future that is based on an institutional willingness to assess the entire information resources of the institution. She proposes guidelines for the future and views these as descriptive, not prescriptive. The one point on which she insists is that the academic health center take a perspective on the entire information resources of the organization and develop strategic planning based on an appropriate information infrastructure. Her view of change in the library profession is in opposition to Bishop when he looks for change over time. She feels that there may be no choice as the revolutionary developments in the transformation of knowledge overtake the library.

The proof of the pudding lay in the tasting. In 1983 the U.S. National Library of Medicine announced a granting program to test the concept of the integrated academic information management model proposed in the Matheson-Cooper report. The objective was to assist the academic medical center in coping with the knowledge explosion and to integrate information management at the institutional level. Four institutions received initial grants to support information management developments that provided for a broad approach to design and gave the necessary financial resources to improve networking and infrastructure, software, and training and education. There was an excitement about these advances in health information integration and delivery that was occurring at these leading-edge institutions and at subsequent institutions that received grants. The process and early results of the experiment in integrated management of information were described in several symposia published in the *Bulletin of the Medical Library Association*.[32]

These innovations were looked on as models by many medical librarians both in the United States and abroad. But the implementation of comprehensive Integrated Academic Information Management Systems, as these specific programs were known, was a very costly undertaking and required a continuing commitment to sustaining the benefits of the integrated planning. Values continued to unite medical librarians, but a gap was growing between the advanced and well-funded health libraries and others that were less well developed or resourced. And that gap was not limited to librarians in the developing world.

International Medical Librarianship in the 1980s

The same environmental factors that provoked the Matheson-Cooper report and the Integrated Academic Information Management System program of grants from the U.S. National Library of Medicine were at work in other countries. The stimulation of international exchange, the increasing reliance on information technology, and a sense of mission stimulated medical librarians to resurrect the idea of an international congress on medical libraries. Following a hiatus of twelve years, the Fourth International Congress on Medical Librarianship was convened, the first congress to be held in a Communist country; earlier congresses had been held in London, Washington, and Amsterdam. The choice of Belgrade as the conference site for the fourth meeting in 1980 suggests an openness and an interest in medical libraries outside of Western Europe and North America. We shall see how the broadening of this perspective continued in subsequent congresses and remains into the present, the ninth congress in Brazil in 2005. The meeting in Belgrade, Yugoslavia, in September 1980 had a significant impact on international medical librarianship for a number of reasons, moving structured international cooperation from a reactive to a dynamic position by ensuring continuity. The Fourth International Congress on Medical Librarianship also issued a planning document, a departure from earlier congresses.[33]

This was an ambitious document, emphasizing the important contribution to the delivery of health care that the medical library could play. Regrettably, this contribution was not always recognized by other health care professionals who often failed to see the medical librarian as a full member of the health care team. This statement was more or less true in the developed world, and there were few medical librarians from the developing world who would dispute it. The report issued a number of strong, far-reaching resolutions on the education and training of medical librarians worldwide, the development of resources in medical libraries, and information transfer between the developing and the developed world. Linking the role of medical libraries to the goal of the World Health Organization, "health for all by the year 2000," the recommendations from the 1980 meeting stressed the role that medical information could play in achieving the goal of health for all. Reading these resolutions today, one realizes how many of these goals have yet to be achieved. Like the WHO goal of health for all, much remains to be accomplished, despite the significant progress that has been made. What had been resolved echoes, waiting for future generations to achieve. The resolutions were designed to guarantee a momentum of change and cooperation that had been revitalized in Belgrade after a gap of twelve years between meetings. Irwin Pizer, who chaired the Drafting Committee, created the necessary dialogue with the International Federation of Library Associations and Institutions (IFLA) that made it possible for the IFLA Section on Medical and Biological Sciences Libraries to serve as a coordinating agency for future congresses. Pizer had also been instrumental in persuading the IFLA executive to create this section a few years earlier. As a result of the acceptance of this role by IFLA, congresses would be held at regular intervals of approximately five years and the planning of these meetings would have a permanent home. The 375 medical librarians from around the world who assembled in Belgrade in 1980 may have been ambitious in their goals, but they certainly were pragmatic in ensuring that a continuing dialogue among medical librarians worldwide would occur. Thus far, the congresses have been held at regular intervals, thanks to the Pizer initiative.

In 1985, the Fifth International Congress took place in Tokyo, Japan, with 567 medical librarians in attendance and the theme "Medical Libraries—One World: Resources, Cooperation, Services."[34] There was great interest on the part of the delegates in developments at the U.S. National Library of Medicine and, in particular, the work being done in the Integrated Academic Information Management Systems program.

The impact of the U.S. National Library of Medicine upon the development of medical libraries worldwide cannot be overemphasized. Over the years, in fulfilling its national mandate to serve the American people, it has opened the world of medical libraries to new methods of control, access, and management of medical information, while remaining a national institution. The Canadian situation in the mid-1980s serves as an example of this impact and the support that was being provided. Elmer Smith, director of the Canada Institute for Scientific and Technical Information (CISTI), formerly the National Science Library of Canada, at the time recognized this vital contribution on the international scene.[35] Smith sees the establishment of a Health Sciences Resource Centre (HSRC) at CISTI directly as a result of a consultation visit by a team of Canadian medical librarians to the U.S. National Library of Medicine in the mid-1960s. Unfortunately, in 2005, this center no longer exists at CISTI. CISTI had become a MEDLARS center in 1970, originally as an off-line literature-search service with a turnaround time between two and three weeks. In 1972, it went online with MED-

LINE. Canadian medical librarians had been aggressive in their demands to provide this online access in part because of the strong and well-established links with American medical librarians through the Medical Library Association. They saw what was taking place in American medical libraries and were determined to make the same improvements in access to medical information available in Canada. By 1986, 300 MEDLARS centers were available in Canada, thanks to the collaboration between CISTI and the U.S. National Library of Medicine. This pattern in growth of use of MEDLARS service was to be repeated worldwide during the 1980s. Smith takes note of these developments and speaks glowingly of the collaborative development of the MEDLARS database.

> In 1985 about 39 percent of the articles indexed for *Index Medicus* were provided by non-U.S. centers, either through their own indexing or through paid indexing done by the U.S. contractor. As other countries were consulted on the control of the Index, they came to feel that it was, in a very real sense, theirs. This in turn has led to what is called the MEDLARS family.[36]

Smith notes that indexing for MEDLINE in countries outside the United States required that MEDLARS countries have a service infrastructure in place. This requirement encouraged countries around the world to invest in appropriate information infrastructure and services if they wished to provide MEDLARS service. In part III of this book we shall see how this ensured world of a MEDLARS community worldwide, where foreign partners were extensions of the National Library of Medicine, has been profoundly altered. But in the world of the 1980s it was very much a consolidated and controlled world of medical information delivery.

In 1986, the year in which the National Library of Medicine celebrated its sesquicentennial, the library could take pride in its international achievements, for it had partnered with institutions in fifteen other countries as well as the World Health Organization and the Pan American Health Organization to form a network of public institutions that had become far more than a means of making MEDLARS available in other countries. These countries were helping to formulate policy and to develop the international network that would be responsible for the dissemination of medical information worldwide. The National Library of Medicine provided further support through its Special Foreign Currency Program, which provided funding for foreign medical publications and translations in partnership countries. The long-range plan of the library done in its sesquicentennial year reaffirmed these international initiatives.[37]

The revitalization of international medical librarianship in the 1980s also gave rise to another formative development: in 1986 cooperation among European medical librarians was strengthened by the first European Conference on Medical Libraries. In a dynamic, emerging unified Europe, the Commission of European Communities and the World Health Organization cosponsored this conference. One of the major impacts of this meeting was the creation of the European Association of Health Libraries. Representation in this new association was taken from the twenty-one member countries, the Council of Europe. From the beginning, the association planned to extend membership to countries outside the original twenty-one members. The unification of European medical librarians in a pan-European association was to strengthen as years passed, and the quality of papers presented at meetings was to increase, as subsequent years demonstrate. A review of the proceedings of this first meeting although not of the meeting itself, was not flattering and says more about profit margins in publishing than about the congress:

> As would be expected of an international conference, the quality of papers ran the gamut from highly sophisticated accounts of state-of-the-art technologies to rather dull "this is how we did do it/show and tell" papers. The physical appearance of the published volume is a disappointment. While the binding and quality of paper stock were of an acceptable standard the camera-ready-copy offset printing technique used by the publisher resulted in a distressing variety of mismatched type fonts and irregular format styles. Because the publisher chose not to do any editing there is an abundance of typographical errors; the use of non-standard English grammar is common. The retail price of $107.50 seems over-priced, a perfect example to fuel the concern that U.S. librarians have over the high pricing policies of European publishers. Given this excessive price and the nature of the volume's content, this publication will have little relevance for the small hospital and most medical school libraries. Large medical school libraries with international programs, library science school libraries, and libraries already with a standing order to the series may wish to add it to their collections.[38]

This review may appear harsh, given this was the first meeting, and it is unlikely that there was much infrastructure in place for paper review and editing. Probably there was a desire to include as many representative papers as possible. However, the criticism that this volume caused due to its price was yet another demonstration of the challenge of paying the bills that librarians had to confront. This problem is dealt with more fully in future chapters of this volume. Here it is interesting to note that it was the medical library profession, with the assistance of the publisher, that had created the problem.

NOTES

1. Scott Adams, *Medical Bibliography in an Age of Discontinuity* (Chicago: Medical Library Association, 1981).

2. U.S. National Library of Medicine, *Classification: A Scheme for the Shelf Arrangement of Books in the Field of Medicine and its Related Sciences*, 2nd ed. (Washington, DC: Govt. Print. Office, 1956), 314; U.S. National Library of Medicine, *Medical Subject Headings*, 1st ed. (Washington, DC: Government Printing Office, 1960), 356.

3. "The National Library of Medicine Index Mechanization Project," *Bulletin of the Medical Library Association* 49, no. 1, Part II (January 1961): 1–96.

4. L. T. Morton, "Notes from London," *Bulletin of the Medical Library Association* 49, no. 2 (April 1961): 210.

5. Keyes D. Metcalf, "Housing the Library, Part I: The Old Building," *Bulletin of the Medical Library Association* 49, no. 3 (July 1961): 396–402; Walter H. J. Kilham, "Housing the Library, Part II: The Old Building," *Bulletin of the Medical Library Association* 49, no. 3 (July 1961): 403–10.

6. Beatrice Simon, *Library Support of Medical Education and Research in Canada* (Ottawa: Association of Canadian Medical Colleges, 1964).

7. MEDLARS is the acronym of the U.S. National Library of Medicine's "Medical Literature Analysis and Retrieval System," which emerged with the mechanization of *Index Medicus* in 1962. It included MEDLINE, the best known of its products and many other specialized databases and services.

8. Simon, *Library Support of Medical Education and Research in Canada*, 70.

9. Hilda I. MacLean, "National Services Provided by the Health Sciences Resource Centre of Canada," *Bulletin of the Medical Library Association* 58, no. 3 (July 1970): 341–45.

10. Alan M. Rees, "Medical School Libraries, 1961–1971," *Bulletin of the Medical Library Association*, Suppl. 60, no. 2 (April 1972): 1–13.

11. Martin M. Cummings and Mary E. Corning, "The Medical Library Assistance Act: An Analysis of the NLM Extramural Programs, 1965–1970," *Bulletin of the Medical Library Association* 59, no. 3 (July 1971): 385–86.

12. Susan Crawford, ed., "Health Sciences Libraries in the United States: A Statistical Profile," *Bulletin of the Medical Library Association*, Suppl. 60, no. 2 (April 1972): 1–56.

13. Joan Titley Adams, ed., "Health Sciences Libraries," *Library Trends* 23, no. 1 (July 1974): 3–175.

14. Mildred C. Langner, "User and User Services in Health Sciences Libraries: 1946–1965," in J. T. Adams, "Health Sciences Libraries," 8.

15. Louise Darling, "Changes in Information Delivery," *Library Trends*, in J. T. Adams, "Health Sciences Libraries," 32.

16. "UCLA Develops Center Serials Control System," *Bulletin of the Medical Library Association* 59, no. 3 (July 1971): 524.

17. Glenn Brudvig, "The Development of a Library Minicomputer System: The Minnesota Experience," *Automated Activities in Health Sciences Libraries* 1, no. 2 (1975): 13–17.

18. Rolf Weitzel, "MEDLINE Services to the Developing Countries," *Bulletin of the Medical Library Association* 64, no. 1 (January 1976): 32–35.

19. Estelle Brodman, "Medical Libraries around the World," *Bulletin of the Medical Library Association* 59 no. 2 (April 1971): 227–28.

20. Estelle Brodman, "The Delivery of Medical Information in the 1970s" (keynote address, Conference on Medical Libraries, Dallas, Texas, Feb. 18–19, 1971), *Bulletin of the Medical Library Association* 59, no. 4 (October 1971): 582.

21. Wyndham D. Miles, *A History of the National Library of Medicine, the Nation's Treasure of Medical Knowledge* (NIH Publication No. 82-1904) (Washington, DC: Government Printing Office, 1982), 456.

22. Miles, *History of the National Library of Medicine*, 457.

23. Helen Crawford, "In Search of an Ethic of Medical Librarianship," *Bulletin of the Medical Library Association* 66, no. 3 (July 1978): 334.

24. Crawford, "In Search of an Ethic of Medical Librarianship," 335.

25. Crawford, "In Search of an Ethic of Medical Librarianship," 336.

26. Crawford "In Search of an Ethic of Medical Librarianship," 336.

27. Nina W. Matheson and John A. D. Cooper, "Academic Information in the Academic Health Sciences Center: Roles for the Library in Information Management," *Journal of Medical Education* 57, no. 10, Part 2 (1982): 1–93.

28. Matheson and Cooper, "Academic Information in the Academic Health Sciences Center," 6.

29. Nina W. Matheson, "Perspectives on Academic Health Sciences Libraries in the 1980s: Indicators from a Delphi Study," *Bulletin of the Medical Library Association* 70, no. 1 (January 1982): 28–49.

30. Matheson, "Delphi Study," 1982, 48.

31. David Bishop, "Testing the Model: Some Reflections on the Matheson Report," *Bulletin of the Medical Library Association* 72, no. 1 (January 1984): 31–32 and Nina M. Matheson, "The Author Replies: Neither True nor False, but More or Less Useful," *Bulletin of the Medical Library Association* 72, no. 1 (January 1984): 32–34.

32. "Symposium on Academic Information in the Academic Health Sciences Center: Roles for the Library in Information Management," *Bulletin of the Medical Library Association* 71, no. 4 (October 1983): 404–34; and Naomi Broering, ed., "Symposium: Integrated Academic Information Management Systems," *Bulletin of the Medical Library Association* 74, no. 3 (July 1986): 235–61.

33. "Fourth International Congress on Medical Librarianship, Belgrade, Yugoslavia, Report of the Drafting Committee on Plans for the Future, September 4, 1980," *Bulletin of the Medical Library Association* 69, no. 2 (April 1981): 263–67.

34. "Special Repsort: Fifth International Congress on Medical Librarianship, Tokyo, Japan, Sept. 30–Oct 4, 1985," *Bulletin of the Medical Library Association* 74, no. 3 (July 1986): 265–66.

35. Elmer V. Smith and Florentia Scott Janson, "Exporting the American (Information) Revolution: The International Impact of the National Library of Medicine," *Bulletin of the Medical Library Association* 74, no. 4 (October 1986): 339–43.

36. Smith and Janson, "Exporting the American (Information) Revolution," 342.

37. Richard K. C. Hsieh, "International Programs of the National Library of Medicine," *Bulletin of the Medical Library Association* 76, no. 1 (January 1988): 54–57.

38. [Review of Patrick W. Brennan, *Cooperation and New Technologies*], *Bulletin of the Medical Library Association* 76, no. 2 (April 1988): 190–91.

III

MEDICAL LIBRARIES IN THE AGE OF THE INTERNET

6

DIGITIZATION AND THE INTERNET:
A REVOLUTIONARY CONTEXT
FOR LIBRARIES

THE COMMUNICATIONS
REVOLUTION IN HISTORIC CONTEXT

Really significant technical revolutions are not very difficult to spot. The historical record readily displays a large number of reactions to the emergence of the printing press, all demonstrating the same point: people were totally aware that "something big" was happening. But a clear perception and consensus on the significance of the events was not present. At an early stage, many people came to realize that the new technology of printing did not simply limit itself to fulfilling its ostensible function—namely multiplying copies at a dizzying rate. Printing was changing many rules and means of control. Who could print? What could be printed? How should it be stored, circulated, made accessible? In effect, a technical solution to the production of texts turned out to be the basis for an entirely new system of communication, and that new system of communication had somehow to be fitted within complex social communities, each with its unique power structure, rules, and traditions. If truly revolutionary, the technical solution is—in fact must be—a source of perturbation as well. However, social structures, institutions, and ultimately people do not like being unduly disrupted. Mentioning the name of Martin Luther is probably sufficient in this context. Luther's use of the printing press is famous for the way in which it allowed him to subvert a great deal of the Church's power. Ironically, the Church had initially extolled and embraced the new technology, and done so quite enthusiastically. Little had it understood that printing could also bolster the gravest danger it ever faced, the ability to make available large numbers of copies of alternatives to accepted Catholic doctrine.

Today, not only libraries but societies are in the midst of an information revolution equivalent in significance to that of Gutenberg and his colleagues. For the past sixty years, people have grown ever more conscious of the ever more pervasive importance of information technology and communications. They may call it "computers" rather than "digitization," but they really mean digitization. The technology that started with mammoth machines that cost an arm and a leg, even from the military perspective, is now available on the desk of millions of people. When computers were big, locked in specially cooled rooms, attended to by a clergy of computer scientists wearing white lab coats and closely watched as should be the case with very precious instruments, the future looked as though it were under control. The request not to "fold, spindle, or mutilate" was designed to protect computer punched cards, but it came to be used derisively by students in universities who did not want to fight in Vietnam. Computers went mini at about the same time that skirts did, except that the term was far more accurate in the latter case than in the former: a minicomputer in the 1960s and early 1970s, such as a typical Vax machine, still needed a fair section of a good size room. It is in the midst of this "mini" craze, in 1968 to be precise, that a truly visionary psychologist came out with an astute analysis: the computer, according to Joseph C. R. "Lick" Licklider (1915–1990), was not so much a computing machine as it is a communication device. Licklider's paper boldly stated "In a few years, men will be able to communicate more effectively through a machine than face to face."[1] In effect, Licklider was playing Luther to the computer, recasting its functions and social role in ways that had never been initially envisioned.

We have seen in preceding chapters that by the 1960s, computers were becoming truly important for libraries. Being able to create large catalogs of objects and retrieving them fast was an early and obvious application of computers. Quite rapidly, computers were adopted for cataloging and bibliographic tasks, but also in the invention of new tasks. During this period too, Eugene Garfield began tracing citation links from one scientific article to another article, taking his inspiration from a much earlier legal bibliography, *Shepherd's Law Index*. However, these developments, important as they were for scientific communication, were fundamentally a question of applying the computer to text analysis. By contrast, Licklider had understood that the computer could become a genuine communication tool. This point is crucial: if, as they should, libraries are viewed essentially as a communication device thanks to the ways in which they handle large quantities of printed materials, then it is easy to understand that putting a new communication tool on top of the earlier one is bound to create some interesting multiplicative effects. Writing in the 1970s, Louise Darling obviously was thinking along these lines as well when she predicted the future of the medical library, "The goal, as this writer interprets the sign posts along the way, is the gradual conversion of the health sciences library into a communications center working actively with information materials of all kinds, close at hand or distant, for health professions users in the community as well as in the institution."[2]

THREATS, POLITICS, AND THE REVOLUTION IN INFORMATION TECHNOLOGY

In 1958, in the wake of the panic in the U.S. government induced by the Soviet launch of Sputnik, the president's Science Advisory Committee had set up a panel on scientific information under the chairmanship of William O. Baker. In the same period of time, Senator Hubert Humphrey, who was then president of the Senate Subcommittee on Reorganization and International Organization, had been agitating in favor of the creation of a Department of Science. However, the executive branch, under both President Eisenhower and President Kennedy, resisted the idea, and the president's science advisor, Jerome Wiesner, used the time-honored strategy of responding to Hubert Humphrey's pressure tactics through the creation of a committee. The committee was chaired by Alvin M. Weinberg, then director of Oak Ridge National Laboratories. William Baker also sat on this committee, as did Joshua Lederberg, a Nobel Prize winner, who would strongly support Eugene Garfield's attempts to create *Science Citation Index* a few years later.[3] In January 1963, the committee published its report, *Science, Government and Information: The Responsibilities of the Technical Community and the Government in the Transfer of Information*. Hubert Humphrey's dream of a Science Department had been artfully whittled down to an acknowledgement of governmental responsibilities in ensuring adequate access to scientific information, and it had taken five years.

This report should not be dismissed as mere skillful political quagmire production. Reflecting twenty-five years later in his Joseph Leiter Lecture at the annual meeting of the Medical Library Association, Alvin M. Weinberg suggested that the report had managed to touch upon a number of points, among which the following two appeared quite salient: the handling of scientific information ought to be an integral part of science; and retrieval of information must be distinguished from the retrieval of documents. Both statements were extremely profound in their implications. In the first thesis, for example, we can hear the beginnings of the argument that science publishing is part and parcel of the full cycle of a scientific research project. Mark Wall-port of the Wellcome Trust was saying much the same when he declared, in July 2004, to be precise: "The dissemination of research is a marginal cost and part of the costs of research itself."[4] This statement was included in a spirited defense of open access as seen from the Wellcome Trust's perspective. The second point—distinguishing document retrieval from information retrieval—lies at the heart of ideas such as "knowledge broker" or "problem identifier." These and synonymous terms have been increasingly used in the last ten years. The concept of the informationist in clinical medical information is a more recent example of the need to emphasize the content of a document and not the document per se.

The revolution in information communications and technology provided the conditions that would make possible a true revolution in scholarly communication. For example, it is difficult to envision how open access would be possible without the presence of a thoroughly digital context. It is important to note that the spirit in which the computer networks were developed and ultimately emerged, particularly the Internet, which turned out to supersede all other networks, contributed to the growth of an open culture predicated on free communication. With regard to scientific communication, the availability of computers and networks seems to have been noticed first in the 1960s, particularly in institutions supporting scientific research, for example the National Science Foundation (NSF) in the United States. Scientific societies such as the American Psychological Association (APA) also studied scientific communication in roughly the same period.[5] Clearly, the Cold War provided the context and impetus for such investigations, as science and technology were viewed as essential resources in this global contest. But matters of fiscal efficiency also emerged as a consideration. The quest for the best "bang for the buck" extended to scientific communication. Out of these "national security" concerns came the verdict that the journal system was far from optimal, even disregarding cost considerations—another issue that also began to reemerge in the 1970s. Communication among scientists had to improve and, to this end, various solutions were suggested: for example, creating a central database of articles as well as other experiments in the distribution of articles, including preprints.

Physicists, an essential component of the nuclear armaments race, felt the need at an early stage to improve access and rapid delivery of research results in this strategic area. The Stanford Linear Accelerator Center (SLAC) began to collect preprints in a systematic fashion under the acronym of SPIRES (Stanford Physics Information REtrieval System) as early as 1968.[6]

In many ways, SPIRES was doing in paper form what Paul Ginsparg would begin to do in digital form in 1991. What was missing in the 1960s were cheap computers and, more important, a sufficiently developed Internet to make crucial scientific information widely and rapidly available to most physicists.

Much later, in 1979, the U.S. Congress began to study legislation that would permit funding a central "National Periodicals Center"—an idea resisted not only by publishers, as could be expected, but also by some large libraries.[7] Nothing resulted from this congressional effort, but it nonetheless signaled the fact that the visions that were to guide the development of various types of digital depositories at the outset of the twenty-first century had already been clearly identified several decades earlier. In other words, some of the necessary conditions for a revolution in scientific communication had been identified, aired, and discussed much before the advent of an open-access movement could have even been imagined. Not only were some of the basic elements needed to move toward open access clearly expressed early on, but their transposition into the context of computers and networks was also articulated quite early.

J. C. R. Licklider saw the computer as a communication device. He had also begun to see that Vannevar Bush's Memex dream could be implemented far more efficiently with digital technologies than with microfilms and mechanical spoolers. This was one of the major themes of his 1965 volume, *Libraries of the Future*.[8] Licklider had been present in these transformative events from the beginning when, in 1962, he had joined the Information Processing Techniques Office (IPTO) of the Advanced Research Project Agency (ARPA)—a military research agency created as part of the U.S. Department of Defense in 1958 by President Dwight D. Eisenhower. This was another component of Eisenhower's response to the Soviet Union's launch of the first man-made earth satellite, Sputnik. Licklider's role at IPTO was to connect computers together. Networking computers was deemed useful in order to pool dispersed and extremely costly resources and to share data and research results. During this period, research grant applications frequently included requests for computers, which at the time meant machines that cost in the six-figure range. Reinventing the digital wheel became the fashion of the day, so to speak, to the detriment of governmental agencies and their research budgets. Despite all the help the Soviet Union was unwittingly providing through the threat of Sputnik and Soviet scientific dominance, it was becoming clear that the costs were not manageable. Out of this mix of motives came the ARPAnet project, and Licklider was at the heart of it.

ARPAnet was not built under Licklider's direct leadership, yet his influence during the period that he directed ARPA's Division of Information Technology from 1962 to 1964 was unmistakable. Both Robert Taylor and Lawrence Roberts actually supervised the development of ARPAnet. Roberts became the head of IPTO in September 1969, even as the first ARPAnet node went live at UCLA. He had been very impressed by Licklider's vision of a network of computers, a vision he had begun to expound in the early 1960s. The following quotation, an excerpt from a 1963 memo to the "Members and Affiliates of the Intergalactic Computer" at ARPA, provides a flavor of Licklider's thinking:

> If such a network as I envisage nebulously could be brought into operation, we would have at least four large computers, perhaps six or eight small computers, and a great assortment of disc files and magnetic tape units—not to mention the remote consoles and teletype stations—all churning away. It seems easiest to approach this matter from the individual User's point of view—to see what he would like to have, what he might like to do, and then to try to figure out how to make a system within which his requirements can be met.[9]

The intergalactic computer—an echo of Licklider's famous sense of humor—turns out to be somewhat more modest. However, what was involved was no less than teaching computers to speak to each other despite the fact that they might be using different languages and be unaware of the existence of other computers. Licklider is impressive in his remarkable ability to think big, and yet translate his broad vision into very concrete technical solutions to specific problems. Licklider muses about doing some curve-fitting work in his own area of research, psychoacoustics, and discovering that the local tools are insufficient. However, somewhere in the putative network, on some storage disk, there is a wonderful curve-fitting program that would solve all his difficulties. The problem is it is stored on a remote system, in a foreign format, and written in a code the local machine does not even begin to understand. This is the vision that underlies his efforts to conceptualize a network of a variety of hybrid computers (computers that do not recognize other computers simply because they are different) that nonetheless could come together as a communications network.

Time sharing marks a pivotal moment in the history of computing because it takes into consideration a very crucial fact: in human–computer interaction, computers react much faster than human beings. From the perspective of a computer, human beings are exceedingly slow in performing certain tasks. There is very little for the computer to do except sleep while they await instructions from their human masters. When human beings grasped this reality, the consequence was immediate: a computer is nimble enough to speak to several human beings simultaneously, and this would not be detectable by the user. This new theory of computer communications was time sharing. What followed were even more interesting questions in computer communications. Small consoles already existed that allowed keying data in real time into the machine, but the development of the personal computer really became available in 1975 with the MITS Altair 8800, the first small computer released on the market.[10] This computer, advertised in *Popular Electronics*, was creating a demand that signified the beginning of personal computing.

The emergence of ARPAnet has been recounted a number of times. What is important to note here, however, is that its motivation was not simply, or even mainly, an attempt to create a robust control-and-command system of military communication. That Paul Baran's studies at RAND did play a role in the design of ARPAnet cannot be doubted, but other considerations played an even greater role. Among these, the need to share resources, if only to lower costs, was paramount.[11] File sharing or file transfer protocol (FTP) and distance control of machines (Telnet) were very much the result of the quest to get the most out of a set of very costly research grants. It was meant to control the irrepressible appetite of research teams for the exclusive use of expensive computers. Once in place, and this was unexpected, the very presence of the network began to stimulate the search for better communication systems. For example, e-mail had not been incorporated in the original design of ARPAnet, but it had already appeared on time-sharing computers. By 1971, technical specifications began appearing. In March 1972, Ray Tomlinson, the man responsible for the ubiquitous @ sign, wrote programs to exchange mail through computers.[12] But the point here is not to recount the evolution of e-mail; rather, it is to show that with the presence of networks, something that may well be termed a "communications ethos" began to emerge. As computer networks made obvious the incredible efficiency of what has come to be named e-mail, they also contributed to the spirit of communication to pervade all of the network activities. Most early users of the networks were scientists, first computer scientists, and in rapid order physicists and other disciplinary practitioners. As a result, whole scientific communities began to understand the empowering nature of the network and, as they did, they began to clamor for it. Larry Landweber's attempt to open up ARPAnet to his community of researchers in computer science is the best known example of this desire to take advantage of the communication capability provided by computer networks. At the same time, the growth of this desire contributed to keeping the modalities of scientific communication at center stage.

In this context, it is difficult to resist the urge to mention the role Unix played in the development of a communication ethos based on distributing and sharing.[13] Quirks of history too long and complex to recount here, but linked to a famous antitrust suit against ATT, ultimately led many university computer science centers to load the then popular Vax machines with an operating system that was essentially free and open: ATT owned Unix. Unix began to incorporate all the tools needed to create efficient Internet connections in the early 1980s, particularly in the Berkeley Standard Distribution, generally better known by cognoscenti as BSD. Soon many universities in North America, in Europe, and elsewhere, were developing interconnections while using their free and open Unix operating system. Communicating, sharing of tools and expertise, distributed development, all became the expected norm of behavior among Unix users. Unix conferences helped reinforce this spontaneous commitment to a way of behaving that was quickly understood to create a strong win–win context. The lesson was not lost on a number of practicing scientists. The Unix spirit has led not only to peer-to-peer networks among teenagers intent on sharing the latest tunes at the lowest possible cost (while infringing heavily on copyright), but also to trails of thought that ultimately found a concrete implementation in the open-access movement.

This brief foray into early Internet communication demonstrates that the beginnings of open access, both in technology and in cultural behavior, had a fairly long prehistory. When the open-access movement appeared on the scene in 2002, it did not arise in the minds of a few individuals, but had deep roots in technology and in scientific communication. A history of experiments and experience in sharing, collaborating, and optimizing communication, sometimes propelled by military concerns, sometimes energized by generous forms of common sense, had preceded the invention of this new approach to scientific communication.

Three basic components—a carrier, the transfer of files, and a networked personal computer—provided the necessary tools to enrich access to information, not only within the scientific community but to all citizens who possessed these basic requirements. But accessing electronic information via the Internet required organization, a catalog of information. "Archie," an access tool developed at McGill University in Montreal in 1990, was the pioneer tool for electronic archive access. This paradigmatic search engine gave way to more powerful tools—Yahoo, Lycos, and

Google, as the reliability of the Internet grew throughout the 1990s and the volume of content continued to increase. Like many of the revolutions of the 1960s, the revolution in computer and communications technology was to have transformative implications for both scientific communication and the library.

THE COMMUNICATION REVOLUTION IN LIBRARIES

The computer/communications revolution that began with ARPAnet had profound implications for libraries, allowing libraries not only to do things better but also to do new things.

Time sharing and networked computing were important factors in the evolution of the digital library and, as we have seen, Licklider was at the center of these developments. However, he was to play an even more vital role for libraries when in 1962 he accepted the invitation of Verner W. Clapp, director of the Council on Library Resources, to prepare a study on the future of libraries. He took leave from his position as an engineering psychologist at Bolt Beranak and Newman to study the future of libraries in the information age. The resulting report did not so much define steps toward the future as identify what the future might contain. *Libraries of the Future* makes a remarkable contribution to our story of access to information.[14] It is part of the general history of the information revolution in libraries that is made clear by Licklider in his preface when he refers to the much-cited article by Vannevar Bush[15] as the "main external influence that shaped the ideas of this book."[16] Licklider is thinking about machines that think and in doing so is suggesting an entirely new approach to libraries.

Early in his investigation, he identified a fundamental issue regarding information as opposed to the containers of information. He quickly recognized that is was not the containers, the print, paper, words, or sentences that were at the essence but the facts, concepts, principles, and ideas. He refers to the passiveness of the printed page and hypothesizes "a device that will make it easy to transmit information without transporting material and that will not only present information to people but also process it for them."[17] Here he is anticipating nothing less than the thrust of the 1990s to extract the relevant clinical information from the plethora of published research and present it where and when it is needed. Although Licklider did not have medical information in particular in mind, he forecasts the role of the medical librarian in extracting and synthesizing information, especially in response to a clinical information need. He anticipates as well the development of services, including commercial developments, to fill this need. The tools and technologies of the information age—memory systems, fast processors, human-machine interaction, and multiple-access computer systems—as well as basic principles in the organization of information including hierarchical and co-ordinate indexing are explored. For Licklider, they provide a means of both enlarging and focusing the human mind to take advantage of the vast amount of information that was becoming available. It is, he believes, vital to the development of libraries that they introduce "multiple-console computing systems."[18] This visionary and radical redefining of the future of libraries did not have the impact that from today's vantage point it might have had. Speculation on the reasons must include the fact that society was not yet confronted with a full-blown information revolution. The creation of large amounts of digital information and high-speed networks were still in the future. Yet in reading Licklider one senses both the accuracy and persistence of his ideas as well as his role in the creation of the library of the future.

Truly saltatory change in the way libraries provided access to information became a reality only when print was replaced by electronic publishing; a revolution in scholarly communication that took place only in the 1990s, a quarter century after the publication of Licklider's book. Other factors, primarily economic and legal, also came into play, as scholarly communication became fully digital, and the issue of access to information became a controversial issue. The rights of citizens to information produced by government funding and the rights of patients to information regarding their sickness were to become matters of particular concern. The economics of information, already an issue addressed by medical librarians in the 1930s, reemerges as a major crisis in libraries in the information age.

Throughout much of its history, the medical library stood as a symbol of the archival record of medical history, an orderly place in which research and scholarship were conducted. Medical librarians had thoughtfully adjusted their collections and services as print began to be replaced by digital products, beginning in the 1960s with the automation of library catalogs, progressing through a variety of CD-ROM products, and moving from librarian-mediated searching in batch mode to real-time, end-user searching. The library was a changed place, but medical librarians managed to retain the best qualities and attributes of the traditional medical library. So too were the core values of medical librarianship still intact. As medical libraries evolved and the tools of retrieval changed, the *Index Medicus* became MEDLINE and the forty other databases that comprised MEDLARS, but the transition was one that, at least in retrospect, was part of the general development in the use of technology in the library. Change had not yet been truly saltatory, although it is true that in working with medical libraries in the early 1990s change seemed to be the only reality.

The arrival of the Internet and the Web in the library escalated the pace of change and provided both a new set of problems and a great deal of opportunity for the medical librarian. Whether the impact created problems or provided opportunities was determined in large measure by whether the medical librarian was in an active or reactive position with respect to the advancing digital technology. The world of the Internet is not an ordered universe, and in fact has been compared to the early days of the Wild West; it provided a vast, random, and constantly changing world of information that varied dramatically in quality. Medical librarians were vigorous and proactive in their responses to the opportunities provided by Internet developments. In the case of user education for health professionals, consumers, and patients, medical librarians were highly successful in taking initiatives (see chapter 7 on consumer health information). They built upon strong principles of providing access to health information for all who need to use it. The Internet was to provide a powerful tool in this cause, and librarians recognized its value from the beginning. In the case of providing access to the canon of published scientific and medical journals, librarians have been forced into a less proactive, even a reactive stance, through the well-established policies and practices of many large commercial publishers. These two areas, public access to health information and access to the journal literature, converge, as we shall show, on entitlement to the research results of government-supported research initiatives.

In the 1990s the potential to improve the delivery of medical information was a powerful stimulus to the development of high-speed and reliable networks. The fact that Donald A. B. Lindberg was simultaneously director of the National Coordination Office for High Performance Computing and Communications and also director of the National Library of Medicine doubtlessly created a highly symbiotic relationship between computing and medical communications.[19] In March 1993, Lindberg testified before the U.S. Congress regarding the benefits of investment in high-performance computing. He testified regarding the delivery of medical information to heath professionals

> My own institution, the National Library of Medicine, a component of the National Institutes of Health, has been a leader in outreach efforts to make health professionals more effective by educating them about modern information services and by lowering the barriers to access medical information. As an example, the NLM makes available a personal computer program called Grateful Med, which allows a health professional or

researcher to formulate a database search online in the office or home by simply filling in a form displayed on the PC screen. Grateful Med then automatically connects to the NLM computers and transmits the search result to the user's own computer. Over fifty thousand copies of this program have been distributed, and the majority of searches of the NLM databases now are conducted via this user-friendly software. Grateful Med provides access not only to MEDLINE, the NLM's premier biomedical literature database, but also to a growing number of specialized information collections on topics such as AIDS, cancer treatment, bioethics, and toxicology databanks. The system predates NREN but has become much more effective now that many institutions can use these information access systems at the greater resolution and higher speeds that NREN permits. NLM joins NSF in a Medical Connections grant program to provide assistance to medical centers to become connected to the NREN.[20]

The political argument of national defense used earlier to convince the government of the United States to invest in information infrastructure had been superseded, at least in Lindberg's words, by one of medical information access.

As the 1990s progressed it became clear that content was key. The information age was being defined as an age of information access, and the development of a standard for the creation of electronic text was essential. The creation of Standardized General Markup Language (SGML) provided an electronic publication tool that was both simple and powerful. By 1998, the National Center for Supercomputing Applications at the University of Illinois had created a powerful browser, Mosaic, which accessed electronic documents distributed worldwide. Within short order, governments, associations, universities, and individuals were discovering the value of visibility on the Web, and access and browsing were launched, as was a new category of professionals concerned with web design and representation in a globally connected world. Everything from e-trading to cancer cures became immediately accessible. The challenge, as always, was in the content, and guaranteeing that quality content was publicly available.

The challenge of bringing order to electronic information and harnessing the power of the Internet and the Web encouraged the development of many knowledge-access initiatives to which librarians are making significant contributions: library and scholar portals, gateways, standards for electronic text creation, as well as digital preservation. The Internet very quickly became an integral part of medical library operations. Increasingly, medical information was going electronic, and medical librarians and their users were early enthusiasts. One indication of the completeness of this transformation appeared in the *NLM Technical Bulletin* in May 2004.[21] The publication, created by the determination of John Shaw Billings in 1879, was no longer required in printed form. In less than a half century and within the working life of more than one medical librarian, the culture had been transformed. The press release notes the decline in subscriptions to the *Index Medicus* that began slowly with the introduction of MEDLINE in 1971 and dropped abruptly when MEDLINE became freely available over the Internet in 1997. By 2003, the number of subscriptions had fallen to a mere 155 worldwide. Might Nicholson Baker take up the cause of those early printed copies of *Index Medicus* if they appear in the trash bins of medical libraries?

NOTES

1. J. C. R. Licklider, "The Computer as a Communication Device" (originally published in *Science and Technology*, April 1968), http://memex.org/licklider.pdf (accessed May 12, 2005).

2. Louise Darling, "Changes in Information Delivery in Health Sciences Libraries," *Library Trends* 23, no. 1 (July 1974): 57–58.

3. Much of the information above comes from Alvin M. Weinberg, "Science, Government, and Information: 1988 Perspective," *Bulletin of the Medical Library Association* 77, no. 1 (January 1989), which reproduces Weinberg's Joseph Leiter NLM/MLA Lecture, National Library of Medicine, April 7, 1988.

4. Mark Wallport, "Open Access—a Funder's Perspective," presented at the 33rd Liber Conference in Saint Petersburg, June 29–July 2, 2004, http://www.enssib.fr/article.php?id=183&cat=Biblioth%E8que+num%E9rique&id_cat=183 (accessed November 28, 2005).

5. See *Project on Scientific Information Exchange* (1963–1968), vol. 1 Overview Report and Report 19 (1963); vol. 2, Reports 1015 (1965); vol. 3 Reports 1619 (1968) (Washington, DC: American Psychological Association, 1968).

6. Sune Lehman, "Spires on the Building of Science: Complex Networks and Scientific Excellence" (cand. scient. thesis, The Niels Bohr Institute, Copenhagen, Denmark, 2003), 24, http://www.nbi.dk/~lehmann/main.pdf (accessed November 28, 2005).

7. Carol Tenopir and Donald W. King, "Towards Electronic Journals: Realities for Scientists, Librarians and Publishers, Précis of C. Tenopir," *Psycoloquy* 11, no. 084 (2000), http://www.cogsci.ecs.soton.ac.uk/cgi/psyc/newpsy?11.084 (accessed November 28, 2005). For a typical publisher response, see William A. Snyder's letter in the *Bulletin of the Medical Association* 68, no. 1 (January 1980): 76–77. http://www.pubmedcentral.nih.gov/pagerender.fcgi?artid=226423&pageindex=2#page)

(accessed November 28, 2005). Copyright law had been changed in 1976 in the United States. Of related interest is the *Final Report of the National Commission on New Technology Uses of Copyrighted Works* (July 31, 1978). CONTU, as this committee is generally known, was established by Congress and operated between 1975 and 1978. Its mandate was to determine how the Copyright Act of 1976 should address problems emerging from the presence of computers and copying machines, http://digital-law-online.info/CONTU/PDF/index.html (accessed November 28, 2005).

8. J. C. R. Licklider, *Libraries of the Future* (Cambridge, MA: MIT Press, 1965). The same year, Licklider had published "A Report of the Office of Science and Technology Ad Hoc Panel on Scientific and Technical Communications" (ERIC reports, EDD 048 895).

9. See http://packet.cc/files/memo.html. This is part of Lawrence Roberts's personal site (accessed May 12, 2005).

10. Christos J. P. Moschovitis, Hillary Poole, Tami Schuyler, and Theresa M. Senft, *History of the Internet: A Chronology, 1843 to the Present* (Santa Barbara, CA: ABC-CLIO, 1999).

11. See http://www.rand.org/publications/RM/baran.list.html (accessed November 28, 2005).

12. The first was RFC 0196, "Mail Box Protocol," by R. W. Watson, dated July 20, 1971, http://www.multicians.org/thvv/mail-history.html (accessed November 28, 2005). All of the protocol-related issues of ARPAnet, and later of the Internet, are discussed through a system of publication called "Requests for comments," or RFCs.

13. Peter Salus, *A Quarter Century of UNIX* (Boston: Addison Wesley: 1994).

14. Licklider, *Libraries of the Future.*

15. Vannevar Bush, "As We May Think," *Atlantic Monthly* 176 (July, 1945): 101–8. In this much-cited article Bush invents the term "Memex," a device that stored the accumulated records and information that was indexed and linked and could be retrieved for immediate use. This was the prototype of a future of personal digital libraries and miniaturization.

16. Licklider, *Libraries of the Future,* xii.

17. Licklider, *Libraries of the Future,* 6.

18. Licklider, *Libraries of the Future,* 69.

19. The benefits of the joint role played by Donald Lindberg in the medical community as the director of the National Library of Medicine and as the first director of the National Coordinating Office for High Performance Computing and Communications have been pointed out by Edward Shortliffe in two articles: Edward H. Shortliffe, "The Next Generation Internet and Health Care: A Civics Lesson for the Informatics Community," *Proceedings of the American Medical Informatics Assn. Annual Symposium,* no. 2 (1998), and Edward H. Shortliffe, "Networking Health: Learning from Others, Taking the Lead," *Health Affairs* 19, no. 6 (November–December 2000): 2–3.

20. Testimony on High Performance Computing and Communications before the House Committee on Science, Space, and Technology, Subcommittee on Technology, Environment, and Aviation by Donald A. B. Lindberg, March 25, 1993, http://mail2.cni.org?Lists/CNI-Big (accessed November 19, 2005).

21. "Index Medicus to Cease as Print Publication," *NLM Technical Bulletin*, posted May 4, 2004, http://www.nlm.nih.gov/pubs/techbull/mj04/mjo4-im.html (accessed January 14, 2005)

7

CONSUMER AND PATIENT
INFORMATION: CONVERGENCE
ON THE INTERNET

> Just one week ago two patients readily admitted that they could not read
> information given to them. Frequently, when staff members locate re-
> quested information for married couples, one spouse will read aloud to
> the other who struggles with reading. In our workplace, we encounter
> patients daily who cannot read the written health information provided.[1]

These comments from a librarian at a Consumer Health Information
Center express the challenge facing librarians in the delivery of health
information to consumers. The challenge is a Chinese puzzle of nested
boxes: the challenge of literacy, with which this book opened; the challenge
of information literacy; and the challenge of health information literacy.
Health information literacy in itself has two aspects: medical information
literacy for the health care provider and health information literacy for the
consumer of health care. It is clear that all these "literacies" are interrelated,
and in an era of convergence through information technology and communications, the appropriate strategies for turning the curse of illiteracy
into the blessing of literacy will be found in solutions that build upon the
convergence of the needs of all users of medical information. But the focus must be on the particular problem or information need. Literacy requires the ability to read. Health information may be conveyed orally and
pictorially as well as by the written word, if the ability to read is absent.
There is a focused but a limited solution to the particular information need
in this case. The larger burden of illiteracy from which a patient may also
suffer is neglected. But the librarian, struggling to meet the patient's request
for information and recognizing that literacy skills are limited, is not in a
position to address the more general problem of illiteracy. Other strategies
must be employed. The only truly effective solution is the one that relates

to the need for functional literacy, a larger social issue that continues to plague even the most prosperous countries, in which universal access to education exists. Information technology can both threaten and promise in the creation of a more literate society. A computer equipped with good learning tools and Internet access can excite the imagination. But even the simplest search requires a question that must be posed through writing.

HEALTH INFORMATION LITERACY FOR HEALTH PROFESSIONALS AND CONSUMER HEALTH INFORMATION: THE DISTINCTION

The distinction between consumer health information and health information literacy for health professionals must be kept clear in the Internet era since it is increasingly true that the same health information is available to all—professionals, patients, and citizens alike. Health information literacy for professionals usually is provided by medical librarians as a program to enable physicians, dentists, nurses, therapists, and all health professionals to access medical information through an improved awareness of the variety of resources available and the techniques of effective online searching. These programs are offered to students in the health sciences and are increasingly incorporated into the curricula. A basic course offered in a medical library is likely to include searching the MEDLINE database, an explanation of the vocabulary of MeSH (the U.S. National Library of Medicine online subject thesaurus), a review of other biomedical databases and other resources, and information at the local or institutional level regarding accessing resources and the local technical infrastructure.

Consumer health information is the provision of information on the maintenance of health and on disease to patients and their families or to the public at large. In an article on the demand for consumer health information, Deering and Harris have argued that it includes medical instructions to patients, support for medical choices of treatment and other decisions, health education, and maintenance.[2] In the case of patient information, it may include a pamphlet on arthritis or a detailed article on the use of tamoxifin. Using reference interviewing techniques, the medical librarian determines the nature of the information need and the ability of the requester to use the information and the appropriate sources to draw upon. Consumer health information is ubiquitous today. The challenge is to guarantee that this information is available at point of need, current and accurate, and above all, comprehensible by the user.

The Internet gave medical librarians an extraordinary opportunity to improve the provision of health and medical information to patients and the public at large. It also provided new roles for medical librarians in this area. Long before the arrival of the Internet, however, librarians had been engaged in this service, as seen in the work, in particular of Alan Rees. With the arrival of the Internet and Web-based services, librarians were well positioned to advance public access to health information founded on developments in consumer health information that had begun decades earlier. Librarians had a solid conceptual foundation on which to build service to members of the public in search of medical information, but there was also a need to rethink services and to introduce quality standards to deal with the vast array of health information that proliferated on the Internet.

ORIGINS OF CONSUMER HEALTH INFORMATION

The consumer health information movement has a long if erratic history, perhaps best described until the era of the Internet as "many times a bridesmaid but never a bride." There has been an ambiguity in the relationship between the need for consumer health information and the role of the academic health sciences libraries until recently, as we shall show. In some basic way, consumer health information has always been with us. Growing up in Canada, my mother's Bible for expertise in caring for me was *Dafoe's Guidebook for Mothers*.[3] Dafoe had been the physician appointed by the government of Ontario to provide care for the famous Dionne quintuplets, whom the state assumed needed this special protection despite the objection of the father of the five female infants. Decades later, the sad story of the manipulation and decline of these five young people was told to the public. However, in the less well-informed 1940s and 1950s, it was assumed that such an expert pediatrician as Dafoe would have something of value to say to all Canadian mothers. In a similar fashion in the United States, Benjamin Spock had stimulated improved methods in child care for new mothers with his 1945 book, *Baby and Child Care*. Examples such as these may be found by the thousands and they attest to the need of the public to obtain information in their best interest and in the interest of those they love.

Medical librarians attempted to define their role in the provision of consumer health information, and in 1956, the Medical Library Association presented a symposium on service to the lay public during the annual general meeting.[4] The papers presented describe an honest if somewhat guarded attempt to answer the question of the responsibility of the librarian in this area.

They speculate on the services that the medical library should provide to the public and review the services that are presently being given. Two decades later, in the special issue on health sciences libraries in *Library Trends*, Estelle Brodman looked back with a highly critical eye on these papers and on the state of the provision of health information to the public at large

> How far we have come in broadening access to health sciences libraries in these two decades since these words were spoken can be illustrated by the fact that instead of scheming over ways to keep lawyers and hypochondriacs out of health sciences libraries, we are now encouraging junior college students to use the material offered them in medical school libraries.[5]

Reasons for this improvement in the change of attitude on the part of some medical librarians in the availability of health information to the consumer can be seen in the vast social changes of the 1960s and the greater empowerment of the people. The legislation of important entitlements such as access to health services under government programs in many Western countries and the various movements to ensure the rights of specific population groups, such as women and minorities, gave impetus and power to those seeking further information. At the same time, the move toward greater accountability of the medical profession to the people and the evaluation of research in terms of its benefits to society was growing. As we have seen in the writing of Scott Adams, the drive toward mission-oriented research created a demand for demonstrable results. And in the health field, the public was anxious to see results that could impact on their health. Medical librarians embraced the broadening of service to those who had not historically had access to medical information. But service had to be rethought. The history of the consumer health information service movement is filled with the stories of successful local projects that significantly advance access to information to a particular and local group of individuals. Only with the arrival of the Internet and its penetration into society at large could the development of comprehensive programs in access to health information for all who need to use it finally be achieved. Problems of health information literacy, the need for education programs, and the larger social issue of inequality within a society still required solutions, but the major issue of accessing health information had been solved.

In 1992, Alan Rees was invited to give the Medical Library Association's Janet Doe Lecture on the History or Philosophy of Medical Librarianship.[6] Following decades of leadership in the provision of consumer health information, Rees chose in his invited lecture to address the question of the relationship between physicians and their patients. Rees traces a history of that relationship that describes deterioration from a time before advances in technology changed medical diagnosis. He describes as golden the period when physicians relied more on patients to narrate the symptoms of their illnesses. In the United States, a combination of social change, medical technology, the scale of health care delivery systems, and above all, financial considerations, were to change this more intimate relationship. He interprets patient advocacy and informed consent as responding to the patient's loss of trust in a more remote and impersonal health care provider. He sees health information in the hands of the patient as a means of coping with this dilemma. Armed with the right information, patients are better able to work with physicians on complex decisions regarding treatment choice. Increased knowledge on the part of patients will lead to more meaningful involvement in their care, and will also alleviate, at least in part, some of the anxiety that arises in the face of the unknown. Unfortunately, Rees points out, under Medicare "explanation and education are not reimbursable."[7]

Rees sees a new role for the librarian in patient/physician relations. As the rights of patients were established, the role of the librarian in providing patient information has become clarified. Rees acknowledges the benefit of federal funding in helping to define and test ways of delivering patient information. There have been many advances, but further work is needed in the interface between hospital librarians and patient information with an objective of improving the dialogue between patients and their physicians. Rees's 1992 paper anticipates many of the advances of the 1990s in patient and consumer education when he calls for a revision of the mandate of the National Library of Medicine (NLM) to support the needs of the public for information on health and disease. He foresees the progress made by the National Institutes of Health (NIH) and the NLM in providing health information on websites and in MedlinePlus that have gone far in advancing public access to health information. But the issue of communication between physicians and their patients that Rees stressed in his Janet Doe Lecture is still waiting further work. It is clear that further developments will benefit from the involvement of librarians, thanks to their historic role and to their professional values.

Patient information has much to do with the legal requirement of informed consent, but is driven by more than a legal requirement. Librarians, through their professional associations, have codified their responsibilities to themselves and to the library user in documents such as the Library Bill of Rights of the American Library Association. The ALA statement affirms the role and responsibility of all librarians in providing information to meet the needs of all members of the community served by the library.[8] The ALA statement is aimed at censorship and discrimination; at the same time, it lends strong support to the need to provide information to all who need it. In a similar fashion, two position statements by the Canadian Library Association reaffirm the rights of Canadians to access the information they need under the Canadian Bill of Rights and the Canadian Charter of Human Rights.[9] While these statements deal with information in general, they provide solid support for the provision of consumer health information.

Health professionals have drafted their own documents that deal specifically with the entitlement of patients to information on their disease and modalities of treatment. In 1959, the National League for Nursing (U.S.) created a Patients' Bill of Rights, an attempt to guarantee that a patient received necessary information on disease treatment options and their implications in order to make an informed choice. This concept received considerable reinforcement when, in 1975, the American Hospital Association created a Patients' Bill of Rights that became part of the policy statements of state hospital associations. These included the provision that "a patient has the right to and is encouraged to obtain from doctors and other caregivers appropriate, current and understandable information about diagnosis, treatment and prognosis."[10] As positive and proactive as such statements are, they do not have any legal authority. Further impetus came from the work of the American Civil Liberties Union in its effort to codify and clarify the legal entitlements of patients in the United States.[11] In 2002, the Congress of the United States attempted to provide a firm legal basis in the U.S. Patients' Bill of Rights, which addressed the rights of patients to obtain the medical care that they need. It attempted to ensure that both physicians and patients discussed openly the treatment options. All consumers of health care were, it stated, entitled to receive "accurate, easily understood information and some require assistance on making informed health care decisions about their health plans, professionals and facilities."[12] This bill passed in the Senate but not in the House and therefore failed to become law. These documents were built on the well-grounded assumption that an informed individual is better able to work with the physician on determining methods of treatment and will play a more responsible role in recovery. They also were designed to enhance the value of informed consent. They are based on the strong belief that major benefits could be achieved through the provision of medical information to patients and the general public.

Numerous studies and evaluations of consumer health programs have been published and are important in sharing information regarding the establishment of new programs and in the improvement of existing ones.

Evaluations of existing programs also helped to justify the continuation of services in consumer health, since many of the start-up programs had been funded from existing financial resources, as a priority. In the pre-Internet era of the 1970s and 1980s, the literature of medical librarianship records a number of successful programs in health education by librarians.[13] A concern with program evaluation continued to characterize the medical literature into the 1990s.

At the Delaware Academy of Medicine, library staff undertook a study of the impact of the consumer health information service that was provided by the Delaware Academy of Medicine Library, Wilmington, Delaware.[14] The information was still largely paper based, but staff also provided computer searches and photocopies of articles without charge to members of the public. Librarians at the Delaware Academy of Medicine worked with public librarians in the area to provide referral service through training by academy staff in conducting medical reference interviews. Not surprisingly, the study strongly endorsed the service being provided, with the majority of those surveyed indicating a willingness to pay for the service. The Delaware study provided insight into consumer health programs just prior to the availability of MEDLINE on the Internet and the development of MedlinePlus.

Projects in consumer health information and their evaluation were part of many organizations during the pre- and post-Internet era. But they were not part of the programs of all medical libraries. Some librarians did not consider consumer health services as part of their legitimate mandate and were therefore reluctant to allocate resources to this need. Some left the provision of consumer information to other libraries in their region, usually to the hospital library or to the local public library, which may or may not have been equipped to provide this information. The responsibility of the academic medical library in this information chain was not always recognized. There were a number of reasons for this reluctance to step up to the need of the general public for health information. Resources to support public health information varied widely depending upon finances, governance, motivation, and even the physical location of the library. A medical library might develop an active collection of materials in consumer health information, but the dynamic outreach to the public might not exist; more proactive was the work of librarians who developed links on their library sites to websites that provide reliable health information for consumers; a medical library may partner with a public library to promote public access to consumer health information. The response of the medical librarian to the active provision of public health information was not uniform, nor was it uniformly proactive. In 2000 Rees noted that genuine progress had been made when he commented that "as a body, the Medical Library Association (MLA) has moved from skepticism to espousal of consumer health as an integral part of the responsibilities of medical librarians, and now actively promotes information services for medical consumers."[15]

CONSUMER HEALTH
INFORMATION IN THE INTERNET ERA

Clifford Lynch has noted the reservations with which some medical librarians entered into the role of information provider to consumers of health care and to the public at large.

> Historically, many biomedical librarians had little to do with communicating information directly to patients, consumers and families. They provided professional and scholarly information to health care providers and researchers, and the health care providers were responsible for telling the patients what they thought the patients needed to know. To the extent that patients or the public wanted to consult the literature, the public library was left to mediate the process, though it held little of the relevant material from the scholarly literature.[16]

But the Internet era was to change the reluctances that Lynch identified. Even prior to the Internet era, some medical librarians had begun to speculate on new roles in information management and in information outreach programs. The development of library programs in user education in searching the medical literature had greatly expanded since the advent of MEDLINE and these programs were given fresh impetus when unmediated (end user) searching was introduced. As the use of the Internet grew dramatically, librarians became concerned, even stressed, by the amount of unreliable information people were accessing. In trying to introduce order and reliability on behalf of their users, they developed criteria for the evaluation of information as well as links to websites of quality information. In the 1970s and 1980s, prior to the Internet, the provision of health information services was encouraged by federal funding under the National Library of Medicine for programs such as the Community Health Information Network (CHIN) and the Consumer Health Information Program and Services (CHIPS).[17]

The remarkable and rapid developments of telecommunications and the Internet required vision and planning in all libraries. In 1996, the U.S. National Library of Medicine under the leadership of Donald Lindberg convened a Long Range Planning Panel on International Programs. In establishing the panel, the NLM recognized that its international activities had never been studied within its long-range planning cycle and convened a committee of experts to present a report on which future planning could be based. This was a key moment, with the Internet in place and the pace of development in biomedical research and medical information accelerating. The panel consulted broadly and had input from medical librarian consultants who queried medical libraries around the world regarding the NLM's international programs. This visionary exercise foresaw an International Network of Libraries of Medicine. Linked by the Internet, these libraries would form a global consortium, making information available at point of use, wherever it might be. The panel recognized the de facto leadership role the NLM was playing internationally through its products and services. It also recognized the value of having MEDLINE available freely and globally over the Internet. Its recommendations included as a first objective "strengthen and expand global access to the world's health-related literature."[18]

Two major program developments of the NLM, universal availability of the MEDLINE database and the development of the MedlinePlus consumer health database, dramatically altered the nature of patient and consumer health information. In 1997, NLM opened worldwide access to the world's largest database of reference to the medical literature, MEDLINE. This knowledge source, once the domain of the physician, the researcher, and the medical librarian, was accessible now to all—the high school student, the public, and the patient. During the first year of universal availability, use of MEDLINE increased from seven million to more than two hundred million searches. A second major initiative was launched on October 22, 1998, when the NLM gave to the citizens of the United States direct access to a powerful resource for health information in MedlinePlus. "In creating MedlinePlus, NLM uses years of accumulated expertise and technical knowledge to produce an authoritative, reliable consumer health Web site."[19] One of the reasons for its enthusiastic reception was that MedlinePlus addressed the uneven quality of information available on the Internet. The "plus" in MedlinePlus is the information from medical encyclopedias, dictionaries, and reference works, giving details on diagnosis, treatment, and prognosis on more than seven hundred medical conditions. In addition, it provides directories of health professionals, pharmacies, and hospitals in the United States. It also links to other authorities on consumer health resources available on the Internet. Since it was launched, the number of unique visits to this site has grown to eighteen million per quarter.[20] It continues to provide a valued resource for health care consumers, journalists, and professionals as a result of its currency, reliability, and ease of access. MedlinePlus was an instant success. It became the home medical companion of the Internet era and made achievable informed consent and health information for all. By 2004, MedlinePlus had been in existence for six years and Donald Lindberg, director of the NLM, noted that "the success of Medline Plus is a testimonial to the public's thirst for health information that they can trust."[21] Although not part of the publicly oriented MedlinePlus initiative, it is equally important to note that the data in the Human Genome Project is also freely accessible from the National Center for Biotechnology Information, a division of the NLM.[22]

MedlinePlus was accompanied by the growth of a number of other health-oriented websites, some of which have become recognized by medical librarians for their excellence in consumer health information. These include the Medical Library Association, Chicago, which identifies websites of quality; NOAH (New York Online Access to Health), a portal that links to high-quality sites, and the sites of the Harvard Medical School (http://www.hms.harvard.edu) and the U.S. National Cancer Institute (http://www.cancer.gov). The National Network of Librarians of Medicine (U.S.), South Central Region, has prepared an online manual of consumer health issues (http:/nnlm.gov/scr/conhlth/hlthlit.htm). This brief mention of sites is neither definitive nor representative but reflects the increasingly high quality of information available to the public.

These developments illustrate how deeply the rights of patients to health information have become embedded in the values and practice of medical librarians. Librarians are promoting public access to health information "in the public good." In so doing they are encouraging individuals to acquire and understand the information relevant to their personal needs. They are promoting health information literacy through instruction in information technology and by providing critically important information. Helping patients to face complex choices in treatment is at the heart of this information. These are major achievements, but there is no room for complacency. According to a report of the American Medical Association, groups with the highest prevalence of chronic disease and the greatest need for health care were least able to read and comprehend the information needed by patients.[23] Low health care literacy contributes to the likelihood of failure in medical interventions. Consumer health librarians have an important role to play in bridging this divide. They are assured of the strong support of the NLM in this effort. In its Strategic Plan for Addressing Health Disparities, 2004–2008, one of the objectives is improvement in health information delivery through the development of easy-to-use information resources, such as MedlinePlus, that are sensitive to the diversity of cultures, education levels, and languages.[24]

With these developments came the need to ensure that the public at large was able to make the best possible use of MedlinePlus in acquiring the information necessary to maintain and improve health. Immediately following the introduction of MedlinePlus, the NLM began to explore how best to move the information to the public through a project that involved public librarians in providing health information. Since public libraries were mandated to serve the public at large and were increasingly involved in providing Internet access to their communities, it seemed reasonable to involve them in health information outreach. The result was a pilot project, the Public Library Consumer Health Information Project, linking public librarians and medical librarians in the National Network of Medical Libraries. Librarians received development grants and participated in training programs to expand access to health information in local communities.[25] The synergy between the two librarian specialties of public and medical librarianship proved most successful in providing health information on the Internet to the public at large. In 2000, fifty-three consumer health information subcontracts were awarded to medical, hospital, and public libraries in the United States by the National Library of Medicine. These projects focused on the improvement of access to electronic health information, in particular to MedlinePlus. They emphasized the development of teaching and training skills on behalf of the general public and aimed at testing the effectiveness of the information being provided by the NLM. Some of the successful projects focused on information targeted at particular consumer groups—the aged, Native Americans, or groups with an interest in a particular disease such as AIDS or Alzheimer's disease. All were concerned with strengthening consumer health information outreach and shared a common commitment to making medical information available at point of need. They also shared a belief that an informed patient is an empowered patient and that knowledge of health matters can help to improve the quality of life and in the prevention of disease. A strong commitment to collaboration between librarians and in the value of the convergence of expertise was at the heart of the success of this program.

The Health Sciences Library at the University of Illinois at Chicago was one of a number of libraries to receive project grants for health information outreach under this initiative. The particular initiative in this instance involved working with groups in the community rather than with individual libraries to promote access to consumer health information.[26] The goal of the project was the promotion of community health through the improvement of knowledge of the environment in a particular neighborhood. Community members were educated to use the literature of public health and, in turn, to provide information within the community. A number of factors—information readiness, the presence of a librarian or information professional in the target community, and familiarity with that community and contacts in the community—were identified as contributing factors in the success of the project. The collaboration of the university's Health Sciences Library and the Cook County Hospital Department of Family Practice were strong factors in the success of the project to improve quality of life in a particular community through access to information.[27]

Five years after the NLM had made available the grants in support of consumer health outreach projects through the National Network of Libraries of Medicine (NNLM), a comprehensive analysis of these efforts to improve access to health information by consumers appeared in *Library Trends*.[28] These descriptions of state-of-the-art projects in consumer health information across a variety of types of libraries highlight the transformation that has occurred in the availability and distribution of consumer health information over the Internet. They also demonstrate the reinvention of the librarian's role in providing these services to the public. The success of each of the projects and the zeal with which librarians collaborated to improve services and empower users is noteworthy but not surprising. The core values of providing access to information wherever it is needed and the role of the librarian as an educator found the perfect environment in nurturing access to health information on the Internet. The projects highlight the collaboration necessary if consumer health information programs are to be successful. The goal of improving health through access to information is shared not only across various types of libraries and community agencies but also with health planners and governments. Another basic reality demonstrated clearly by these projects is that progress in improvement of health through access to information will be at a local level. Many of the fifty-three projects are targeted to very particular issues or diseases, and the focus is the local community. Programs were sustained once the grant had expired, through the incorporation of the particular consumer health information program into the services of the library, a strong indication of the importance of this service to the community.

SOME DEVELOPMENTS OUTSIDE THE UNITED STATES

The need for consumer health information was being met by librarians in many different settings and countries. Developments in the United Kingdom illustrate the integration of various types of librarianship in the interests of improving public access to health information. Librarians became interested in exploring the information needs of particular health information consumer groups such as the elderly or the hearing disabled.[29] The National Health Service became interested in the issue of consumer health as well, and in 1983 the British Library reviewed the provision of general health information services to the public, as part of its responsibilities under the National Health Planning and Resources Act (1974), which identified health information as a priority.[30] In 1997, the Dearing Report had emphasized that students needed to equip themselves for lifelong learning through the acquisition of information literacy skills.[31] Within the health sector, the National Health Service produced a report in 1999 that emphasized the need for developing skills in information literacy and information management. This stress on information literacy was taken up by the Society of College, National and University Libraries (SCONUL), which in 2001 produced its "Seven Pillars of Information Literacy."[32] Convergence was taking place on two levels. Convergence between general information literacy and health information literacy became a powerful driving force among librarians in general. A second convergence was also taking place between a health-information-literate society and an information-literate health professional.

Other nations were equally concerned to advance the health of citizens by providing public health information over the Internet. In France, Rouen University Hospital launched *Catalogue et Index des Sites Médicaux Francophones* (CISMeF) in 1995, initially as a source guide for health professionals and later as a source of health information for patients and the public at large.[33] Its objective was to provide access to French-language resources using as a means of organization MeSH, the subject thesaurus of the U.S. National Library of Medicine and the Dublin Core metadata format, tools to provide for the international exchange of information through standards. CISMeF was conceived to address the need for French-language health resources and for the cataloging of French-language materials. The use of CISMef reflects this need: 70 percent from France, 16 percent from Canada, especially Quebec, 4 percent from Switzerland and Belgium, and 3 percent from Africa.[34] As CISMeF evolved, it became more consumer and patient oriented. Medical librarians in North America have been known to refer to it as the "French MedlinePlus."[35] Like MedlinePlus, CISMeF includes a list of medical topics and related information. Its creators also share a concern with evaluating its effectiveness by patients and the public who are using it as a source of health information. CISMeF is supported in part by the Government of France Ministry of Research.

In Canada, the use of the Internet to provide health information to the public at large has become part of government planning. The government has created the Canadian Health Network/Reseau Canadien Santé (CHN/RCS), providing health information by groups, topics, and particular diseases. Medical librarians in Canada see a role for themselves in working with the Canadian Health Network to provide quality consumer health information, although this role has not been clarified at the national level.[36] The reason is perhaps not the result of the planning process or the failure to recognize the potential of medical librarians in this area. Rather, it is more likely the result of the perennial Canadian dichotomy between federal and provincial mandates. Both health care and education are matters under the jurisdiction of the provincial governments of Canada's ten provinces. Under these conditions the creation of a national mandate is complex, and more immediate results may be obtained at a local or regional level.

Excellent work in consumer health and patient information is being done at a more local level in a number of Canadian libraries and institutions. Toronto's University Health Network provides professionally validated patient information via its Patient Education Network. This Toronto-based network provides services across three hospital sites and is also Internet accessible.[37] At the provincial government level, for example, the government of Ontario has developed a reliable website and a telephone hotline for public health information.[38] And at the municipal level there are a number of excellent initiatives in place, for example, those offered in major metropolitan centers such as Vancouver and Toronto through the public library system.

Canadians may seek information on health and disease at numerous websites such as those mentioned. They may also use the highly developed and richly resourced site of MedlinePlus and CISMeF depending on their linguistic preferences. But those sites are not Canadian and may not include information on uniquely Canadian issues of health policy and legal matters. Medical librarians both in Canada and elsewhere are likely to direct those seeking health information to quality websites, and not engage in the creation of information, a wise decision—provided that governments, associations, and other agencies have created reliable sites. Canadian medical librarians are analyzing options and modalities for providing coordinated access to information by users seeking patient and consumer health information. The need is certainly a pressing one. A 2003 working document on health information options by James Henderson and Associates speaks about these issues. Henderson quotes the results of a 2003 survey by HealthInsider of Canada, noting that of the 70 percent of Canadians surveyed, more than half (53 percent) were seeking health information.[39] Heavy use of the Internet for health information has been demonstrated repeatedly. Over forty-one million Americans were active users of the Internet in 2000, and it is estimated that half of all usage is health related.[40]

THE ROLE OF THE MEDICAL LIBRARIAN

Given the proactive role of governments and health professionals in providing medical information to the health care consumer, it is important to define the role of the medical librarian in this process. The role encompasses the responsibility for providing information service and the development of health information literacy skills. The Medical Library Association has integrated the provision of health information literacy into its objectives, not surprising given the profession's historic core value of providing access to information and user education. The Association's Task Force on Health Information Literacy has defined health literacy as "the set of abilities needed to recognize a health information need; identify likely information sources and use them to retrieve related information; access the quality of the information and its applicability to a specific situation; and analyze, understand and use the information to make good health decisions."[41] Readers familiar with the definition of information literacy adopted by the Association of College and Research Libraries will note how closely this definition follows that of ACRL.

Health information literacy is a requisite set of skills for both the health professional and the public who seek to inform themselves on matters relating to their health or disease. To work toward the provision of health information literacy for the general public, the Medical Library Association established a Section on Consumer and Patient Health Information, which provides courses for medical librarians, produces a newsletter, and moderates an electronic discussion group. A number of medical librarians active in this section have compiled guides to consumer health information on specific topics. Core bibliographies identify useful reliable information resources that assist librarians in providing answers to specific health-related questions. They also help to establish the resource requirements for a Consumer Health Library. Successful examples of these library-based consumer health services exist. Consumer health and patient information services occur in many different settings: medical libraries, hospital libraries, public libraries, government agencies. They may be paper-based or virtual or a combination of print and electronic resources. And the success of these endeavors appears to increase directly with enhanced collaboration between public and medical libraries and with the integration of the service into the community. The New York Online Access to Health (NOAH) represents a highly successful model, engaging a variety of kinds of libraries—the Library of the New York Academy of Medicine, the New York Public Library, the Library of the City University of New York.

In the Internet era, the provision of health information to the public and the development of health information literacy skills for the public have given exciting new roles to medical librarians. Dealing with the convergence of information sources in an open information environment creates challenges in the organization as well as the interpretation of these resources. It may prove interesting to consider a possible historical parallel to Patients' Libraries in the evolution of consumer health information services and the role of the medical librarian. At one time in the early twentieth century, the idea of a library of reading materials for patients was a dynamic movement led by physicians and librarians. Their work was grounded in a firm but untested belief that reading was therapeutic.[42] The Patients' Library Movement was part of medical librarianship throughout the first half of the twentieth century. Patients' libraries required an organized collection of suitable materials and a professional librarian with formal training and understanding of bibliotherapy. Patients' libraries were usually located in hospitals. They were prominent at the end of World War I and again after World War II ended, suggesting a particular relevance to the needs of wounded veterans. Their presence in hospitals also suggests a period when a patient was well enough to enjoy the therapeutic benefits of reading, but sick enough to stay in hospital. Oh happy middle ground prior to managed medical care!

These libraries were very strongly linked administratively to the doctors' or medical library in the hospital and were, for a number of years, part of the discussion of standards for hospital libraries. The idea of the patients' library in the Internet era suggests an interesting parallel. Patients' libraries, based on the belief in the therapeutic value of reading, received considerable attention in the first half of the twentieth century. Patients' libraries no longer exist, and the reasons for their demise have much to do with the social values of the time. The reasons also may include the reality that those librarians who worked with patients' libraries more than half a century ago did not ask the question: "What difference does this service make?" The assumption that reading improved health was never validated by those who espoused it.

In the Internet era, medical librarians are enthusiastically engaged in the creation of consumer and patient information services, believing, along with many other professionals, that patient information can improve the health and recovery of the patient. One very productive area of research that librarians could pursue more intensely is the proof of the concept that a well-informed patient is more likely to recover from illness and to benefit from medical intervention. Some research is being conducted in this area,[43] but larger-scale and less anecdotal studies are required if this work on behalf of the public is to be funded at an appropriate level. The idea that the right information in the hands of the medical practitioner can save lives is part of the current effort to push clinical medical information to the bedside. But the study of the impact of health information on the patient requires more research better to inform and shape patient information services. Medical librarians can and should make a strong contribution in this research area. They would also find many willing partners. Governments in the developed world are spending millions of dollars on public education in the areas of disease prevention and a healthy lifestyle. Medical librarians engaged in patient and consumer health information are in an ideal position to initiate and to collaborate on studies regarding the extent to which the availability of this information is making a difference.

NOTES

1. Patricia A. Hammon, "Developing a Health Literacy Action Plan," *MLA News*, no. 364 (November 2004).

2. M. J. Deering and J. Harris, "Consumer Health Information Demand and Delivery: Implications for Librarians," *Bulletin of the Medical Library Association* 84 no. 2 (April 1996): 209–16.

3. Allan Roy Dafoe, *Dafoe's Guide Book for Mothers* (Toronto: Smithers, 1936): 246.

4. "Symposium I–V: Service to the Lay Public," *Bulletin of the Medical Library Association* 43, no. 1 (April 1955): 241–62.

5. Estelle Brodman, "Users of Health Sciences Libraries," *Library Trends* 23, no. 1 (July 1974): 64.

6. Alan M. Rees, "Communication in the Physician/Patient Relationship," *Bulletin of the Medical Library Association* 81, no. 1 (January 1992): 1–10.

7. Rees, "Communication in the Physician/Patient Relationship," 3.

8. American Library Association, *Library Bill of Rights* (adopted June 18, 1948 by the ALA Council, amended February 2, 1961, inclusion of age reaffirmed January 23, 1996), http://www.ala.org/ala/oif/statementspols/librarybillrights.htm (accessed March 25, 2006).

9. Canadian Library Association, Statement on Intellectual Freedom (approved by Executive Council, June 17, 1974, amended November 17, 1983 and November 18, 1985), http://www/cla.ca/about/intfreed.htm (accessed March 25, 2006); and Canadian Library Association, Action for Literacy (approved by Executive Council, February 7, 1993, amended June, 1993), http://www.cla.ca/about/literacy.htm (accessed March 25, 2006).

10. See http://www.hospitalguide.mhcc.state.md.us/Misc/patient_bill_of_rights .htm (accessed March 25, 2006).

11. George Annas, *The Rights of Patients: The ACLU Guide to Patients Rights*, 2d ed. (Carbondale: Southern Illinois University Press, 1989).

12. U.S. Senate, McCain-Edwards-Kennedy Patients' Bill of Rights bill S1052, http://democrats.senate.gov/pbr/summary.htm (accessed March 26, 2006).

13. See for example: F. B. Colleen and K. A. Soghikian, "A Health Education Library for Patients," *Health Services Review* 38 (1974): 236–43; D. Eakin, S. J. Jackson, and G. G. Hannigan, "Consumer Health Information: Libraries as Partners," *Bulletin of the Medical Library Association* 68, no. 2 (1980): 220–29; C. L. Harris, "Hospital Based Patient Education Programs and the Role of the Hospital Librarian," *Bulletin of the Medical Library Association* 66, no. 2 (April 1978): 210–17; D. J. Richards, "Providing Health Care Information to Patients in a Small Hospital," *Bulletin of the Medical Library Association* 66, no. 3 (July 1978): 342–45.

14. Victoria Pifalo, Sue Hollander, Cynthia L. Henderson, Pat DeSalvo, and Gail P. Gill, "The Impact of Consumer Health Information Provided by the Libraries: The Delaware Experience," *Bulletin of the Medical Library Association* 85, no. 1 (January 1997): 16–22.

15. Alan M. Rees, *Consumer Health Information Source Book*, 6th ed. (Phoenix, AZ: Oryx Press, 2000), 9.

16. Clifford Lynch, "Medical Libraries, Bioinformatics, and Networked Information: a Coming Convergence," *Bulletin of the Medical Library Association* 87, no. 4 (October 1999): 410.

17. There were two major programs funded in the east (CHIN) and west (CHIPS) of the United States to advance the provision of consumer health information services. See, for example: Ellen Gartenfeld, "Community Health Information Network (CHIN)," in *Developing Consumer Health Information Services*," edited by Alan Rees (New York: Bowker, 1982) and Eleanor Goodchild, "The CHIPS Project: Health Information to Serve the Consumer," *Bulletin of the Medical Library Association* 66, no. 4 (October 1978): 432–36.

18. U.S. National Institutes of Health, National Library of Medicine. Report of the Board of Regents. National Library of Medicine Long Range Plan. *A Global Vision for the National Library of Medicine*, September, 1998. (NIH Publication No. 99-4330)

19. Naomi Miller, Rebecca J. Tyler, and Joyce E. Backus, "MedlinePlus: The National Library of Medicine Brings Quality Information to Health Consumers," *Library Trends* 53, no. 2 (Fall 2004): 375.

20. MedlinePlus, http://www.medlineplus.gov (accessed July 14, 2006).

21. Press release: "MEDLINE Plus Is Six Years Old on October 22," http://www.nlm.nih.gov/news/medplus 6yrs.html (accessed January 15, 2005).

22. Press release: "Public access to the human genome," http://www.nlm.nih.gov.archiv/20040831/news/press-releases/humangenome-pr01.html (accessed January 15, 2005).

23. AMA Council on Scientific Affairs, "Report of an Ad Hoc Committee on Health Literacy." *Journal of the American Medical Association* 281, no. 6 (February 1999): 552–57.

24. U.S. National Library of Medicine, "Strategic Plan for Addressing Health Disparities, 2004–2008," http://www.nlm.nih.gov/pubs/plan/nlm_health_disp_2004_2008.html (accessed September 18, 2004).

25. Fred B. Wood, Becky Lyon, Mary Beth Schell, Pauline Kitendough, Victor H. Cid, and Elliott R. Siegal, "Public Library Consumer Health Information Pilot Project: Results of a National Library of Medicine Evaluation," *Bulletin of the Medical Library Association* 88, no. 4 (October 2000): 314–22.

26. Carol S. Scherrer, "Outreach to Community Organizations: The Next Consumer Health Frontier," *Journal of the Medical Library Association* 90, no. 3 (July 2002): 285–89.

27. The Chicago Environmental Public Health Outreach Project (CEPHOP) website: http://www.uic.edu/depts/lib/projects/resources/Cephop/ (accessed January 20, 2005).

28. "Consumer Health Issues, Trends and Research: Part 1, Strategic Strides toward a Better Future," *Library Trends* 53, no. 2 (Fall 2004); and "Consumer Health Issues, Trends and Research: Part 2, Applicable Research in the 21st Century," *Library Trends* 53, no. 3 (Winter 2005).

29. See, for example: M. J. Rowe, "Information for Health Now, with a Happy Retirement in View," *Health Libraries Review* 1, no. 1 (March 1984): 11–15; Hilary Todd, "The Information Needs of Newly Retired People," *Health Libraries Review* 1, no. 1 (March 1984): 29–35; W. Anderson, "Sleeping Giants: Towards an Understanding of the Needs of Deaf People," *Health Libraries Review* 1, no. 2 (June 1984): 83–87.

30. Elaine Kempson, "Review Article: Consumer Health Information Services," *Health Libraries Review* 1, no. 3 (September 1984): 127–44.

31. "The Dearing Report," formally known as "Reports of the National Committee of Inquiry into Higher Education in the United Kingdom," was published in 1997. Sir Ronald Dearing is the principal author. http:www.leeds.ac.uk/educol/niche/ (accessed July 15, 2006).

32. Margaret Haines and Gary Horrocks, "Health Information Literacy and Higher Education: The King's College London Approach," World Library and Information Congress, 70th IFLA General Conference and Council, Buenos Aires, Argentina, Health and Biosciences Libraries. http://www/ifla.org/IV/ifla70/prog04.htm (accessed January 18, 2005).

33. See http://www.chu-rouen.fr/cismef/ (accessed January 17, 2005).

34. S. J. Darmoni, J. P. Leroy, F. Baudic, M. Dougere, J. Diot, and B. Thirion, "CISMeF: A Structural Health Resource Guide," *Methods of Information in Medicine*, 39 (2000): 30–35.

35. Stefani, Stefan, Benoit Thirion, Sylvie Platel, Magaly Dougere, Philippe Mourouga and Jean-Philippe Leroy, "CISMeF-patient: a French counterpart to MED-LINE plus," *Journal of the Medical Library Association* 90, no. 2 (April 2002): 248–253.

36. See http://www.canadian-health-network.ca/servlet/contentserver (accessed January 18, 2005).

37. See http://www.uhn.ca/patient/health_info/index,asp/bav=2;2 (accessed January 20, 2005).

38. See http://www.HealthyOntario.com (accessed January 20, 2005).

39. "Information on Disease Management and Therapy: Issues and Options for the Canadian Health Network" (Réseau Canadien de la Santé, December 15, 2003, James Henderson and Associates, 2003).

40. Alan M. Rees, ed., *Consumer Health Information Source Book*, 6th ed. (Phoenix Arizona: Oryx Press, 2000), ix.

41. See http://www.mlanet.org/resources/healthlit/ (accessed January 20, 2005).

42. Nancy Mary Panella, "The Patients' Library Movement: An Overview of Early Efforts in the United States to Establish Organized Libraries for Hospital Patients," *Bulletin of the Medical Library Association* 84, no. 1 (January 1996): 52–62.

43. An example of the kind of research that has been undertaken in this area is found in Jane Sweetland, "Users' Perceptions of the Impact of Information Provided by a Consumer Health Information Service: An In-depth Study of Six Users," *Health Libraries Review* 17, no. 2 (June 2000): 77–82.

8

NEW APPROACHES TO CLINICAL
MEDICAL INFORMATION

New and expanded demands by patients for information arose with the arrival of medical information on the Internet. Rees and others have attributed those needs in part to a changing, more litigious and technological era of medical practice. But other causes can be identified. Advances in health care occur daily, informed and improved through new discoveries in medical research. The average life expectancy, at least in the developed world, seems to increase with every report. And the sick, suffering from what once were thought to be mortal diseases, are living longer with their illnesses; some even consider themselves cured. Modern medicine and disease-centered research have made these developments possible. Doctors may be taking less time to listen to their patients and relying more on tests, but more advanced medical tests are providing increasingly reliable information about the hold a particular disease has taken on a particular patient.

Typically, a patient is tested following a general diagnosis based on symptoms identified by a patient during the initial interview with a physician. Tests take the clinical investigation further and validate or negate the hypothesis that the physician made during the initial diagnosis. Modern drug therapies and treatments are powerful, and side effects need to be carefully considered within the context of the individual patient. As the public becomes better informed about the secondary effects of drug therapies, there is an increasing need to justify their use and to explain possible subsidiary effects upon the patient.

With deliberate irony, Richard Horton comments on the shift away from listening to patients, noting that "the experience and feelings of the patient are of marginal importance in making judgments about what treatments to offer. The patient is an obstacle in the consultation rather than a source of critical information."[1]

Having captured the reader's attention with this challenging opinion, Horton argues strongly for a synthesis in medical care combining the best in qualitative and intuitive diagnosis in medicine based on experience, practical knowledge, and careful listening by the consulting physician, with the power of scientific medicine and technology. His final conclusion is a bold and reasoned reversal of his attention-getting original statement, "modern medicine must encourage doctors not only to listen to what patients have to say but to believe it."[2] In passing, he gives further support for systems of patient information, stating, "If patients' expectations are enhanced by providing information about the illness or its treatment, the outcome of that illness can only be substantially improved. Management of patient/doctor relationships can affect the disease process."[3]

Recall the role for hospital librarians advocated by Rees in helping to improve physician/patient communication: Horton is advocating much along the same lines. Richard Horton is a dramatic and confident writer, working through strong convictions on both sides of an argument to arrive at a powerful synthesis. He clearly recognizes the value of medical information and the importance of information literacy in the medical profession, as the following anecdote dramatically illustrates.

> Surgery is all about action, not reflection. But information is sometimes critical, even in the operating room. In 2002, surgeons in Australia were working frantically to save the life of a critically injured man. One of the surgeons recalled that he had read an article in a medical journal that he was sure would help him and his team right there and then. The problem was that he could not remember which article. What could he do? A call was put out to the British Library archives. Although it was received at 3 AM British time, library staffs were able to track down the 1996 paper in the *European Journal of Emergency Medicine* within twenty minutes and send it to the desperate Australian surgeons.[4]

Today, just a few years later, his comments could be viewed as somewhat anachronistic. The field of medical librarianship has been dramatically reengineered to provide even greater access to information at point of need than described in Horton's anecdote. From the organization of document provision to end user open access to information through PubMed and PubMed Central, information is being pushed out to health care providers at point of need, with the majority of these benefits available internationally. Medical librarians have developed new initiatives in using these developments; in fact they have fully redesigned their services and libraries to optimize the delivery of medical information at point of need in the Internet era. Programs in end user searching, evidence-based medicine, and medical informatics are built upon the need to deliver the necessary information where it will do the most good.

DEFINING NEW ROLES IN
CLINICAL INFORMATION DELIVERY

The professional literature of science and medicine available in a well-stocked library or, in the Internet era, at the desk of a user, provides what is arguably the most important continuing education resource. But getting that information to the clinical practitioner precisely when it is most needed and in a readily accessible format is a continuing challenge to the medical librarian. By the early 1990s clinical information delivery had made major advances using a plurality of methods to improve access. These developments had grown out of early efforts such as those of Gertrude Lamb at the Hartford Hospital, Connecticut, and the Literature Attached to the Charts Program (LATCH). The availability of high-quality medical information on the Internet created new roles for the librarian in teaching end user searching. Specialized services to clinicians and specialized clinical resources, particularly databases emphasizing case studies and reports, developed. Clinical medical librarianship emphasized the role of the librarian in the selection and provision of the most appropriate information resources to meet the needs of a particular physician in the treatment of a particular patient. Training the user of information or "end user training" was concerned with helping the clinician to search highly specialized clinical information resources. It had been clear for decades that clinicians had distinct and different information needs from the medical research community, and meeting the needs of this particular segment of the user community had become a strong specialization within the general practice of medical librarianship.[5]

Medical librarians were finding new opportunities to express their values and purpose in the Internet era and were becoming key players in the growth area of providing health information to patients, their families, and the general public, as seen in the work of Alan Rees and his successors. The vision of their future was being recast by the Medical Library Association in emphasizing the value of librarians as providers of quality information to improve health. The vision statement of the association "Professionals Providing Quality Information to Improve Health" placed no boundaries on the delivery of quality information by medical librarians. Users of medical information resources may be health professionals, patients, or consumers, in fact, anyone who requires information regarding a health issue. Medical librarianship is transformed in the information age, but at the same time its core values are being reasserted. This reinterpretation of the perennial values of the profession in the information age has been described by a past president of the Medical Library Association, Michael Homan:

> Although the core values and vision remain unchanged, MLA is now facing some of its greatest threats and potentially most rewarding opportunities. A central theme in both these threats and opportunities is the changing profession and the need for health sciences librarians to build on the past and reengineer themselves to meet the information-intensive demand of health care for the future.[6]

When medical librarianship became more patient centered, it was responding to the changes in the teaching and the practice of medicine. Medical librarians quickly adopted the role of educator of health care professionals in providing them with the necessary skills in health information literacy to search the literature and to access information in an increasingly digital and networked world. And this role of providing access to health professionals to support patient care has an ever increasing possibility of being extended to include patients, their families, and the general public as part of the community of health-information users. However, the skills and the information are not always the same, although both activities follow from Homan's reengineering of the role of the medical librarian.

How best to provide this information to the patient and the consumer is the concern of the consumer health librarian, as described in chapter 7. But could not these services also be provided by the clinical medical librarian, bearing in mind that health information literacy for the patient is a different matter from health information literacy for clinicians? Librarians have more than three decades of experience in providing information through programs in clinical medical librarianship. The intent of clinical medical librarianship from the beginning has been the improved use of medical information in a clinical setting. Clinical medical librarianship (CML) took the librarian out of the library into the clinical setting to become involved in patient rounds, to improve speed and access to information directly related to specific clinical situations. Librarians became the information component of the health care team in the treatment of a particular patient. Clinical medical librarians were the original data miners in health information, unlocking the vast storehouse of medical information in medical libraries, and selecting only the most highly relevant materials. The potential for more effective use of the time physicians spent in reviewing the literature was a subsidiary goal. The early days of CML paralleled the early days of the digital medical library. Library automation was in place, but networks for delivering that information were not robust or well developed, and searching on remote host computers where the medical information resided was done by librarians rather than the end user. As described in chapter 7, demands of patients for information regarding their illness and choice of treatments had yet to be fully articulated and given complete legal sanction. Programs in CML spread rapidly through the medical library community, and a period of evaluation followed that included studies of the impact of these programs on the information needs of physicians and other members of the health care team.[7]

Following several decades of experience with programs in clinical medical information, Wagner and Byrd published a study of the effectiveness studies that had been done on programs in CML.[8] Using the published literature that reviewed a variety of CML programs over time, the authors analyzed surveys and data regarding particular programs better to understand their effectiveness. Many of the studies described particular programs and individual institutions while others such as the Rochester Study[9] looked at a broad range of studies. Wagner and Byrd found in their review that while all programs were perceived as having a positive impact, there was very little evidence to support the hypothesis that the information provided through CML services contributed directly to improved patient care or better performance by the health care professional. It is important to read carefully the findings of Wagner and Byrd since existing CML programs could be influenced by their conclusions. Their review of the literature of CML failed to identify significant direct, measurable relationships between information availability and clinical outcomes. However, there appears to be significant evidence that is qualitative, anecdotal, and supported by user surveys in many evaluation studies on the perceived usefulness of the information provided in CML programs. Wagner and Byrd call for further study of the outcomes on patient care, length of stay in hospital, mortality rates, and so on in conjunction with programs in CML. They further note that the anecdotal evidence is overwhelmingly positive. The only negative reported by a health care team member who had worked with a clinical medical librarian was the lack of time in which to read the medical information that had been provided. This criticism speaks to health care management issues rather than to CML programs. The authors conclude that

the total amount of research evidence for CML program effectiveness is not great and most of it is descriptive rather than comparative or

analytically qualitative. Standards are needed to consistent¹y evaluate
CML or informationist programs in the future. A carefully structured
multiprogramme study including three to five of the best programs is
needed to define the true value of theses services.[10]

The potential to view the discussion of Wagner and Byrd as critical of
CML must be avoided; their work criticizes the evaluation process by failing to quantify patient-centered outcomes—not an easy task. Does the
right information at the right time help to save lives? Many medical librarians entered the profession with this sense of mission. One medical librarian has put it this way in describing what he will say to an introductory class
in medical librarianship: "I am going to make the point that what makes
our specialty different from all of our librarian colleagues is literally a matter of life and death. At the end of the day, this is what ties us together as
health sciences librarians."[11]

But can it be proven that a particular piece of information at a specific
time helped to save a particular human life? Billions of dollars are spent annually based on the importance and necessity of medical information systems and delivery. In any evaluation, context and timing play a role second
to the design of the evaluation. And the Wagner and Byrd study appeared
when a new form of medical information professional was being debated:
the health informationist. In an editorial that appeared in the *Annals of Internal Medicine*, Davidoff and Florance, a physician and a librarian, discussed
the reasons that a new kind of health information professional, the informationist, was needed.[12]

Before looking at the implications of this seminal concept, it is helpful to examine the conditions that made possible its development. The
teaching and practice of clinical medicine was evolving through a series of
major new initiatives, problem-based medicine and evidence-based medicine, and an increasingly patient-centered system of health care. As these
concepts were incorporated into medical education and clinical problem
solving, medical librarians reengineered their programs and services in an
effort to respond better to new curricula. In fact, these developments also
shaped clinical medical librarianship.

Of equal importance to the changing role of the medical library had
been the advent of end user searching, strongly advanced and promoted
through the Grateful Med program of the U.S. National Library of Medicine that had been launched in 1986. Grateful Med was designed to sim-
plify searching of the medical literature directly by physicians and other
health care personnel. By the late 1990s programs in end user searching and

clinical medical librarianship proliferated and had been in place for a sufficiently long time to be evaluated seriously. It was time to take a close look at the success of these programs in improving physician access to the medical literature. In addition, the 1990s had seen the arrival of databases such as UpToDate and the Cochrane Databases of Systematic Reviews. These electronic services were derived from the primary medical literature and extracted medical best practices and specific clinical therapies and results in a synoptic fashion with an objective of improving ease and speed of access to medical information. These developments seemed to suggest that the time-honored method of searching and retrieving the quality-filtered information in the primary literature in medical databases such as MEDLINE was not the most effective way of providing clinical medical information. These new syntheses of clinical medical information in evidence-based databases recognized the reality that the medical literature had become so vast and the clinicians' time so limited that new solutions were needed.

These recent developments suggested that further review of the effectiveness of CML programs was necessary, although there was a ready acknowledgment that these programs has been providing quality information-filtering services. One of these studies[13] was done in the early 1990s at the Hospital where Gertrude Lamb had launched the pioneer program in CML in 1973 as director of the Health Sciences Library at Hartford Hospital, Connecticut. This single case study is representative of many similar evaluations that were to be cited in the Wagner and Byrd review of CML programs. The point is that this review occurred at the hospital where CML had been born. The author of the Hartford study concludes that based on admittedly limited evidence and despite advances in end user searching, the program in CML at Hartford Hospital "continues to provide information that directly and indirectly affects patient care."[14] The conclusion is nuanced, stating that "for the present" the program has not been displaced by end user searching. The need for further research is clearly imbedded in the author's conclusions.

The Davidoff and Florance idea of an informationist is born at the end of a long decade that witnessed the greatest revolution in scholarly communication and publication since the Gutenberg era. It was conceived in a climate that repeatedly stressed the need for evaluation, effectiveness, and cost containment. It is grounded in the requirement of all physicians to base their clinical decisions on the most reliable precedents in clinical practice. The authors acknowledge that despite the extraordinary efforts of the U.S. National Library of Medicine and many medical librarians to promote the use of Grateful Med, the literature is not being used as effectively as possible. In fact, it appears that in making clinical decisions, physicians continue to rely heavily upon the time-honored method of consulting respected colleagues. In the opinion of the authors, the response of medical librarians in creating CML programs has been valuable, efficient, and effective. In reaching this conclusion they cite a number of the same studies as the Wagner and Byrd analysis of CML programs. But despite the acknowledged value of the programs in CML, the authors conclude that CML has not been effectively integrated into mainstream medical librarianship. The reasons for this failure go beyond many of the variables under the control of the medical librarian and result from the shortsightedness of the financial policies that govern health funding.

> Although the current U.S. Medical care nonsystem happily continues to pay billions of dollars for the information generated by millions of inappropriate and unnecessary clinical tests, it unfortunately refuses to pay a dime specifically to move the rich, sophisticated knowledge from the medical literature to the bedside where it might not only improve medical care but might actually save money. The resulting chronic and increasing budgetary constraints on medical libraries mean that vital on-site library staff can't be replaced if they are shifted into clinical services. Even worse, these perverse priorities have resulted in the complete elimination of many hospitals' medical librarians in an effort to "cut waste."[15]

Since, as the authors conclude, CML programs have not been fully developed for financial and other reasons, and since they believe that most physicians do not and should not retrieve the information themselves, the authors advocate for a new national program, modeled on CML, to educate medical information specialists or "informationists," who would be the clinical knowledge workers, analogous to clinical epidemiologists, and would assume roles on the clinical staff of hospitals. The emphasis is on training and credentialing with the candidates eligible for informationist training coming from backgrounds in information and clinical medicine. In the fullest sense, informationists become part of the health care team reporting to health care directors and paid by health care budgets. Launching a demonstration project to test the informationist concept is advocated.

More than five years have passed since the editorial by Davidoff and Florance introduced the concept of the informationist. The impact of this short piece on medical librarians has been extraordinary. In fact, to someone outside of the United States, the subsequent actions represent the American action orientation, the "just do it" philosophy of the United States with strong emphasis on testing and evaluation. Moving from idea to action as quickly as possible without a long-term commitment characterizes this approach, which has been highly successful. In August 2002, the U.S. National Library of Medicine and the Medical Library Association sponsored a conference to explore the informationist concept as a means of improving the use of clinical information. In a thoughtful editorial, T. Scott Plutchak, editor of the *Journal of the Medical Library Association*, described this conference and reviewed possible outcomes.[16] He raised the question of CML programs and their relation to informationist programs; doubtlessly those CML programs that are well established and effective will continue. The Long-range Plan of the U.S. National Library of Medicine had established a goal of strengthening the information infrastructure for biomedicine and health and an objective of training in medical information and librarianship.[17] Exploring the idea of the role and training for informationists fell well within the scope of these goals, and the funding for educational programs became available. The Medical Library Association began to explore the concept as well, launching a project to identify what distinguishes an informationist from a librarian.[18] This study was undertaken with Vanderbilt University Eskind Biomedical Library, where a highly successful clinical information outreach was providing a model approach.

What will be the end result? It is likely that this idea is yet another step in an iterative process that began decades earlier in an attempt to improve access to necessary information by clinicians. It reflects the efforts to relocate the role of the medical library in a changing library landscape and to respond to changing needs using the latest information technologies. As clinical investigation makes more results available more rapidly, the opportunity to improve health through improving access to the results of that information increases. The problem here, as in many areas of scientific investigation, is important, familiar, and not yet fully solved—knowledge transfer. Even with some of the revolutionary tools in information access that are available to the practitioner, such as Grateful Med, open access to an increasing amount of the medical literature made available on PubMed Central and end user search engines designed for the nonexpert medical searcher, the information is not moving adequately from the bench to the bedside or from the published literature to the information problem.

THE U.S. NATIONAL LIBRARY OF MEDICINE—PROVIDING INFORMATION AT POINT OF NEED

The National Library of Medicine has been assisting medical librarians in their role of information provider since the first printed index to the national collection appeared. It has at the same time acted as a powerful support in the delivery of medical information worldwide. It has been helping medical libraries to cope with the volume, costs, and variability in the quality of medical information since its earliest days. In turn, medical libraries have worked with the National Medical Library as advisers and consultants to represent the needs of users and institutions, although relationships between medical librarians and their national resource have been troubled on more than one occasion.[19] On the whole, however, efforts on both parts have made the delivery of services a spectacular success, one that is looked upon at times with envy by librarians working in other countries. The Regional Medical Library Program and its successor, the National Network of Libraries of Medicine, have been a model of service and management that has been emulated in other countries. Most important, the products, the databases of citations, texts, and data, have become part of the work of medical librarians throughout the world. The ripple effect of these products internationally is clear to all who use them.

The decade of the 1980s saw strong penetration of personal computers into the research and medical communities and Internet developments that brought enhanced access to research centers and universities. In 1985, under the leadership of Donald Lindberg, the U.S. National Library of Medicine had launched an improved document delivery service to promote access to the journal literature. DOCLINE, as this program was called, had some modifications and was applied in a Canadian setting as well. One year later, Grateful Med, a software interface designed for MEDLINE searching by physicians who were not trained literature searchers, was launched. Enthusiastically, the National Library marketed Grateful Med directly to hospital administrators, ignoring any mention or communication with the hospital librarians. The voices of medical librarians that were raised regarding this oversight were both unified and strong, especially among hospital librarians, who were already feeling threats of hospital downsizing for financial reasons and library closings. Advocating on behalf of its membership is an important role for the executive and board of any professional association, and the Medical Library Association is no exception. The board of directors acted promptly to point out to the National Library of Medicine its oversight on behalf of hospital librarians by bypassing this component of the association's members, approximately half of whom were hospital librarians.

Two statements published back-to-back in the *Bulletin of the Medical Library Association* by Donald Lindberg and Herbert S. White, distinguished professor, School of Library and Information Studies, Indiana University, capture the nature of the debate.[20] Lindberg's piece stressed the mandate of the library given to it by the Congress of the United States to improve and extend to the rural and underresourced parts of the country the services and products of the library. He emphasized the potential of Grateful Med in helping the library to fulfill this mandate. The need to make available to all citizens the latest advances in health care as presented in the literature of medicine will be served by outreach programs. While recognizing the superior searching ability of many medical librarians who are able to provide answers to complex information questions through mediated searching, Lindberg notes that many of the information needs of clinicians do not represent complex medical searches. Health professionals are able, he feels, to search sufficiently effectively to satisfy their needs for this kind of information. Lindberg also provides a strong definition for the medical librarian's role in the changing information landscape:

> I believe that the role of the health sciences librarian in the 1990's is to be recognized throughout his or her institution as an authority on access to information related to the biosciences. This means having specialized knowledge about the many databases available and the various forms and routes of access. To be recognized as such an authority means knowing about software programs that are used to access, display and reformat the results of a database search. It means having a grasp of the rapidly emerging world of much more powerful systems.[21]

On the other side, Herbert White reasserts a more traditional approach to the role of the medical librarian, deploring the idea of believing medical information can be exchanged without the intervention of the medical librarian. He does not mince words: "Medical librarians need to get out the message that using Grateful Med on your own, in the hope of performing an adequate and cost effective search is not only dumb, it is a dangerous idea." White finds it paradoxical that it is medical librarians on whom the National Library of Medicine must draw in teaching the use of Grateful Med to end users.[22] This debate has historical interest today. White's comments have succumbed to history; in the intervening years medical librarians have embraced a new role of educational specialist in providing health information literacy and searching training to medical school students and physicians. They have capitalized on the changing role of the medical librarian to promote their enduring values of providing access to information and promoting information literacy in the information age. They have moved into new roles as information managers in their institution in providing pathways to accessing increasingly sophisticated systems, as Donald Lindberg's comments presaged.

Internet extension and its increasing reliability provided a powerful new tool for making available the information services of the National Library of Medicine. To better understand how these services could be made available and to use its grants program strategically, the library conducted a survey just as use of the Internet was exploding. It showed some important trends in Internet use and Web-based services. Among numerous other findings, the survey revealed that three-quarters of the NLM users who had Internet access were using it to access the World Wide Web, but less than 26 percent were using the Internet to access NLM databases.[23] The high proportion of users who had Internet access suggested the importance of using it to deliver the information that the library was making available. Internet access was increasing dramatically and promised the possibility of equalizing services to the rural and information-poor areas. These statistics are based on the United States, but the implication of their analysis for providing medical information worldwide will not be missed. The survey also made it clear that scientists, rather than health care providers or librarians, had greater Internet access and higher-end computer equipment. The library's granting programs in support of training, equipment, and demonstration programs were important as a means of extending further access to the library's resources to the health care community. One of the more disturbing findings of the study was that librarians who comprised the most intensive user group of NLM databases had the least effective technical resources (computers and Internet access). This reinforced the importance of the outreach programs and activities of the National Network of Libraries of Medicine. Much of this information had been familiar to librarians working in the field for some time, and they too were concerned to reach the end user who could apply the information on the clinical setting.[24]

But was end user searching by clinicians using Grateful Med the best way to meet this need? In some cases, but certainly it was not the "silver bullet" for the delivery of clinical medical information to physicians at point of need. Grateful Med and Lonesome Doc delivered over the Internet to health care professionals provided a powerful cocktail. Yet despite the efforts of medical librarians and the U.S. National Library of Medicine, there was still an unmet need to deliver information to the bedside of the patient. The majority of intended end users, it appears, were being introduced to these information services, but after the introductory sessions, many were not asking for more.[25]

Health care professionals were participating in Grateful Med training programs in all parts of the United States, with participants given training and a copy of the Grateful Med software, free search time in the era of pre-MEDLINE on the Internet, a number of free articles in DOCLINE as well as consulting and follow-up service. There were many reasons why these programs did not succeed fully in changing the information-seeking behavior of health care professionals. Clinical physicians were constantly aware of time in their patient-filled days. Where were they going to find the necessary minutes to integrate into their daily schedules the need to search the medical literature? This was the concern of some. Others felt that technical difficulties did not merit the time required to overcome them. This reason was likely to disappear for most practicing physicians with the arrival of more stable and rapid communication systems, simpler operating systems, and more robust hardware. A more fundamental issue was continued reliance on traditional methods of obtaining information, such as colleagues or a single source like *PDR* or a textbook. In this case, the introduction of online use of medical information needs to be viewed as a powerful adjunct to these time-honored methods of obtaining information related to patient care.

Perhaps the most significant reality that was emerging was that clinicians appeared to need a synthesis of the required information from a variety of articles, a sort of information bottom line, before they were willing to modify their habits. The need was for highly relevant extracts from an article, not for a number of articles. The concern was the communication of the information itself, not its container, the document. For more than a century the focus of medical librarians had been retrieval and document provision, a role strongly supported through the databases of the literature and the rich and comprehensive collections of the National Library of Medicine. But, at least for some clinicians, it would appear that this was a necessary but not a sufficient condition for bringing information to the bedside. The shift from a citation/source approach to a case-oriented synthesis was significant: it relied upon the literature, but it took the information a step further. This information-on-demand would be designed to provide specific answers to clinical questions.

SYNTHESIZING MEDICAL INFORMATION THROUGH EVIDENCE-BASED MEDICINE

A number of physicians and other health professionals had been considering the question of synthesis of information for some time. In fact it was a natural outcome of the identification of best practices. It also related to a patient-centered approach and emphasized information related to a unique patient. Evidence-based medicine (EBM) takes health information literacy a step further. EBM is the conscientious explicit and judicious use of current best evidence in making decisions about the care of individual patients. The practice of evidence-based medicine requires the integration of individual clinical expertise with the best available external clinical evidence from systematic research and the patient's unique values and circumstances. The work being done at the New York Academy of Medicine in conjunction with the American College of Physicians in developing an Evidence-based Medicine Resource Center serves an example of the application of EBM. The center provides training, resources, and technology to both physicians and librarians in EBM, fostering cooperation between librarians and practitioners to advance the use of evidence-based medical practice. The definition of EBM according to their center is "a methodology for evaluating the validity of research in medicine and applying the results to the care of individual patients. Evidence is gathered through the systematic review of the literature and is critically appraised. The results are integrated with physician/patient decision-making."[26] The importance of EBM, and this is particularly evident in the second definition, is that it is intensively patient centered.

EBM evolved for a number of reasons. Above all, it is an attempt to help the clinician stay abreast of the exponential growth in the amount of medical information, any part of which may contain essential information for the treatment of a particular patient. It is a highly effective and immediate alternative to more traditional ways of staying current, such as visits from pharmaceutical representatives, occasional Continuing Medical Education courses, or browsing journals, either in the library or through personal subscriptions. It often includes criteria for the evaluation of published clinical findings. Teaching EBM is enhanced by certain databases such as the Cochrane Library providing systematic, up-to-date reviews of randomized controlled clinical trials. Some of the databases, such as the National Library of Medicine's MEDLINE, that are part of EBM are freely available to all over the Internet. Others, such as the Cochrane Library, are proprietary. Is the public good being served in these cases? It has been argued that certain databases are not relevant since they require expert knowledge to understand and use them. This may or may not be the case; however, a category of "expert patient" is emerging, as a concerned patient representative. From the international perspective, the important reality is that databases and other information freely available over the Internet can be accessed in the developing world in the interests of promoting "health for all."

NOTES

1. Richard Horton, *Health Wars: On the Global Front Lines of Modern Medicine* (New York: New York Review of Books, 2003), 52.

2. Horton, *Health Wars*, 59.

3. Horton, *Health Wars*, 60.

4. Horton, *Health Wars*, 433.

5. An excellent summary of developments in clinical information services is to be found in Joanne G. Marshall, "Issues in Clinical Information Delivery," in "Libraries and Information Services in the Health Sciences," ed. Prudence W. Dalrymple, special issue *Library Trends* 42, no. 1 (Summer 1993): 83–107.

6. Michael J. Homan and Julie J. McGowan, "The Medical Library Association: Promoting New Roles for Health Information Professionals," *Journal of the Medical Library Association* 90, no. 1 (January 2002): 81.

7. See, for example, P. O'Connor, "Determining the Impact of Health Library Services on Patient Care: A Review of the Literature," *Health Info Library Journal* 19, no. 1 (2002): 1–13; D. N. King, "The Contribution of Hospital Library Information Services to Clinical Care: A Study of Eight Hospitals," *Bulletin of the Medical Library Association* 75, no. 4 (October 1987): 291–301; Joanne G. Marshall, "The Impact of the Hospital Librarian on Clinical Decision Making: The Rochester Study," *Bulletin of the Medical Library Association* 80, no. 2 (April 1992): 169–78.

8. Kay Cimpel Wagner and Gary D. Byrd, "Evaluating the Effectiveness of Clinical Medical Librarians' Programs: A Systematic Review of the Literature," *Journal of the Medical Library Association* 92, no. 1 (January 2004): 1–20.

9. Marshall, "The Rochester Study."

10. Wagner and Byrd, "Evaluating the Effectiveness of Clinical Medical Librarian Programs," 6.

11. T. Scott Plutchak, "Editorial: The Informationist—Two Years Later," *Journal of the Medical Library Association* 90, no. 4 (October 2002): 369.

12. Frank Davidoff and Valerie Florance, "The Informationist: A New Health Profession?" [editorial], *Annals of Internal Medicine* 132, no. 12 (June 20, 2000): 996–98.

13. Robert J. Veenstra, "Clinical Medical Librarian Impact on Patient Care: A One Year Analysis," *Bulletin of the Medical Library Association* 80, no. 1 (January 1992): 19–22.

14. Veenstra, "Clinical Medical Librarian Impact on Patient Care," 21.

15. Davidoff and Florance, "The Informationist," 998.

16. Plutchak, "Editorial: The Informationist—Two Years Later."

17. U.S. National Institutes of Health National Library of Medicine, Long-range Plan 2000–2005, http://www.nlm.nih.gov/pubs.plan/lrp00/goal-3-2.html (accessed January 31, 2005).

18. See http://www.MLANET.org/research/informationist (accessed January 31, 2005).

19. Betsy L. Humphreys, "Adjusting to Progress: Interactions between the National Library of Medicine and Health Sciences Librarians, 1961–2001," *Journal of the Medical Library Association* 90, no. 1 (January 2002): 4–20.

20. Donald A. B. Lindberg, "The National Library of Medicine and Its Role," *Bulletin of the Medical Library Association* 81, no. 1 (January 1993): 71–73 and Herbert S. White, "The Grateful Med Program and the Medical Library Profession," 81, no. 1 (January 1993): 73–75.

21. Lindberg, "The National Library of Medicine," 72.

22. White, "The Grateful Med Program," 75.

23. Fred B. Wood, Karen T. Wallingford, and Elliott R. Siegal, "Transitioning to the Internet," *Bulletin of the Medical Library Association* 85, no. 4 (October 1997): 331–40.

24. See, for example, Cheryl Dee, "Information Needs of the Rural Physician: A Descriptive Study," *Bulletin of the Medical Library Association* 81, no. 3 (July 1993): 259–64.

25. Judy F. Burnham and Michael Perry, "Promotion of Health Information Access via GRATEFUL MED and LONESOME DOC: Why Isn't It Working?" *Bulletin of the Medical Library Association* 84, no. 4 (October 1996): 498–504.

26. Website of the New York Academy of Medicine, http://ww.ebmny.org/thecentr2.html (accessed September 17, 2004).

IV

IS THERE A BETTER WAY?

9

THE ECONOMICS OF SCIENTIFIC
AND MEDICAL INFORMATION

Gaining control of the literature of science and medicine developed
along two separate but related tracks that may be broadly classified as
economic and bibliographic. Economic control includes the acquisition and
creation of journals and subsequently the merger of commercial publishing
houses to create large holding companies. Bibliographic control includes
achieving effective means of organizing and accessing the medical and scientific literature. There are many overlaps in this dichotomy since enormous financial implications result from the invention of bibliographic control systems and the publishing of the scientific literature that is controlled
by private companies. This chapter focuses on the economics of medical
and scientific publishing, the impact of commercial publishing on the library, and one particular attempt, the creation of the "Big Deal," to cope
with the rising costs of the journal literature. The following chapters discuss efforts to develop new ways of providing access to the results of research in science and medicine through publishing outside the dominant
commercial model of scientific publishing.

PAYING THE BILLS: THE EMERGING PROBLEM

In the letters to the editor in the *Bulletin of the Medical Library Association*,
1989, Peter Stangl, the director of the Lane Medical Library at Stanford
University, informed readers that he had sent letters to Elsevier, Springer,
Pergamon, Dekker, Liss, and Karger addressing the very serious issue of
journal price increases.[1] Stangl's gentle admonition on journal costs anticipated a debate that was to be persistent and at times acrimonious, and continues to the present. Stangl urged those to whom he sent the open letter

to begin a dialogue in order to preserve the viability of scientific journal publishing in the face of increases in publication costs. Recognizing that even the wealthiest libraries were unable to meet the high costs of journal materials, he concludes that the only alternative will be the cancellation of journal titles. His argument "that the elasticity of the library market is being exceeded by cost increases" although novel at the time, resonates to the present. He argues compellingly that the present system of scholarly communication must undergo fundamental change if it is to survive. Further, the members of the scientific scholarly community will not themselves be the agents of the necessary change.

The responses from the representatives of several of the publishers to whom Stangl wrote are included along with Stangl's letter. Elsevier's director of Marketing Services, John Tagler, replied in full agreement with Stangl's point that there exists a "long-term need for journal publishing and, by extension, scientific communication to undergo some fundamental changes,"[2] although he regrets that solutions have not, as yet, emerged. Currency exchange rates at the time—the value of the American dollar against the Dutch guilder in which Elsevier journals were priced—is offered as the main reason for major price fluctuations, and Tagler offers hope for the forthcoming year due to the recent stabilization of the U.S. dollar. Thomas Karger of S. Karger, Basel, Switzerland, replies in a similar vein, noting, like John Tagler, the devaluation of the U.S. dollar as a major factor in the price of journals, and promises no increases in subscription costs. Neither the Elsevier or Karger responses discuss the question of profit margins, although a third respondent, Alan R. Liss, Scientific Medical and Scholarly Publications, does mention the fact that his firm does not make enormous profits from journal publishing. This statement is not quantified, but Liss notes that "if we don't make any profit at all we would stop all together and where would you—the user—be then?" Liss's response is still relevant today as it points out the burden librarians continue to carry to the present:

> The journal isn't science, the journal is the message. It is the message that this particular array of information is of scientific importance and excitement. . . . We as publishers can only do our best to help by sifting out the material that is presented to us for publication, by trying to put it in its most useful form which includes rigorous reviewing as well as careful reproduction and preparation. Those are our functions as publishers. *Your function as a librarian extends to arranging that the published material is available in libraries for consultation by those people to whom it is addressed.* It seems to be that the problem lies with woefully insufficient

funding of the library community. The publishers don't create the problem any more than the manufacturers of typewriters do. I suppose I should be more modern and say the manufacturers of computers—they don't create the problem either. The problem comes from the vitality of the scientific and academic endeavor and its output in the form of carefully written, carefully thought out reports of research.[3]

In many ways, the arguments are too familiar. Liss's response is quoted in full as he gives an indication, albeit unwittingly, of the solution to the pricing problem identified in Stangl's open letter. The computer, according to Liss, is not the problem, but it was to offer a solution, one that would become the subject of intense debate a decade later—open access.

The behemoth of journal pricing was beginning, as the Stangl correspondence demonstrates. The crisis provoked anxiety for all librarians, although librarians working in science, technology, and medicine would feel most strongly the impact of aggressive pricing. Understanding the origin of the problem in the system of scholarly communications that extended over centuries was an essential step. It was equally important to comprehend fully the way copyright protection in scientific journal publication acted as a linchpin in maintaining control over pricing and distribution. Returning to the analogy contained in the classic work of Garrett Hardin on shared resources in the commons (discussed in chapter 1, see page 6), librarians were becoming aware of the extraordinary financial consequences of commercial pricing practices and beginning to appreciate that this was a problem for the scholarly community, not only for the librarian community. Achieving the engagement and commitment of the scholarly community in the resolution of the issue continues to occupy the efforts of many librarians. For the scholarly community to engage, researchers needed to understand the issue and accept the fact that the system was no longer functioning. Added to this volatile situation was the determination of librarians to serve their particular community or user group at all costs, that is, at the cost of increasing demands on the university or hospital global budget. The building of strong, comprehensive collections of information required that the necessary information be purchased, *at all costs*. The nature of investigative research made it impossible for a researcher to determine what article or book might be needed, and this omnivorous demand encouraged, if not mandated, comprehensive collections. Of course, the provision of access to information identified earlier as a core value of the library profession was thwarted by cost increases. Anxiety regarding the ability of librarians to provide information was the norm, directly proportional to the increased cost of the journal literature.[4]

The dialog on cost increases initiated by Peter Stangl in the pages of *Bulletin of the Medical Library Association* was the beginning of a quest for solutions and a genuine desire to communicate with the medical publishing world. Concern over the issue of the economics of journal pricing was not uniformly viewed as the most fundamental problem by some medical librarians. Acceptance of some form of "regulated greed" as a way of librarian life was advocated by more than one librarian. Lelde B. Gilman argues that access to information is not at a crossroads since the scientific community in the United States has access to an enormous amount of information.[5] The argument is deflected to the issue of a changing society. It is, according to Gilman, not the scholarly communication process that is the issue; it is the university, and, indeed, the entire society that is in jeopardy:

> The very purpose and mission of the university in a democratic society is currently being debated; the quality of education is in crisis; the education of a physician is currently under scrutiny as being inadequate to meet tomorrow's needs; health care procedures for the poor are being examined and ranked according to who gets what based on cost per benefit for the most; the costs of AIDS and crack are becoming apparent; emergency rooms are closing around the country; and 50 million Americans cannot afford health insurance. Yet we librarians still talk of scientific information as being an inalienable right, of a kinder, gentler world of scholarly publishing; we assume that all can work together for the common good and call for the cooperation of publishers, scientists, scholars and librarians *as if all of us had the same needs or goals.*[6]

The argument that follows this bleak description that normalizes the crisis in scholarly journal pricing rests on distinguishing between the values of librarians, scientists, and publishers. Simply put, librarians want to provide everything to everyone, scientists would like to be right, and publishers want to make money. This simplistic analysis would, naturally, not allow for nuanced discussion, or the development of improved dialogue and understanding of the issues. In fact, it would be foolish even to try. The solution, according to Gilman, was for health sciences librarians to develop more finely tuned, selected collections and define their needs more precisely. This was, of course, exactly what many librarians tried to do in response to the escalation of costs. The issues raised in the Stangl/Gilman correspondence during the early 1990s were repeated frequently at conferences and in institutional settings and were without resolution. In fact, a compromise solution was most unlikely, given the conflicting motives of librarians and for-profit publishers. As the 1990s progressed, the problem of journal price inflation became increasingly challenging in all libraries. By the end of the decade, a full-blown crisis existed.

Librarians in most countries around the world, and especially those involved in the delivery of scientific and medical information and in paying the bills, found reinforcement in the commonality of the problem and in a host of studies on the cost of journals by both government and librarians. Governments were concerned for a number of reasons: the need for a country to maintain a competitive position on the world stage in the information age, the increasingly high costs of doing research and providing financial support to libraries for the information infrastructure necessary to the education and research, and the need for greater public accountability. Governments saw themselves as the ultimate bill payers and took an increasing interest in, among other issues, the cost of maintaining libraries. In the United Kingdom, as early as 1993, a report of the Higher Education Funding Council brought librarians and government together in the writing of the Follett Report. This study was concerned with making the libraries serving higher education in Britain as effective as possible and not in particular with the economics of journal subscriptions. However, it did not shy away from the essential problem of the impact of journal costs on paying the bills.

> In the last decade, there has been a disproportionate increase in the price of books and periodicals, and the volume of publications, especially periodicals. . . . Between 1980–81 and 1991–92 the Blackwell's Periodical Price index rose by almost 300 per cent, library spending within HE institutions on periodicals rose on average only by 111 per cent and the RPI by even less, 71 per cent. . . . These trends have intensified in the last two years with continuing substantial increases in periodical prices and in the prices of specialist monographs. The prospect for 1994 is even worse.[7]

The report resulted in additional funding as well as encouragement toward intensified cooperation and new directions for libraries serving higher education in the United Kingdom, its primary interest and achievement. But it also foreshadowed the important investigations by the government a decade later on the economics of commercial publishing and access to the scientific literature.

In the United States, the Council on Library Resources provided a grant to the Association of Research Libraries in 1986 to study management practices in the nation's research libraries. Martin Cummings, former director of the U.S. National Library of Medicine, was engaged to review management practices in the nation's research libraries. Cummings produced a solid study on the economics of research libraries and thus provided an improved understanding of the costs of resources required by the library. His work, like the Follett report, was designed to improve library management, but we see again the growing concern with the costs of library materials:

> The materials themselves have been increasing rapidly in price. The average U.S. hardcover book cost $5.24 in 1961 and in 1982 cost $25.48, a 309 percent increase. The cost of U.S. periodicals increased 438 percent in the same period and the average increase for all materials was 365 percent or about 17 percent per year.[8]

Cummings identifies a number of now familiar strategies for coping with this reality: cancellation of duplicate subscriptions, increased library resource sharing and interlibrary loan, diminishing the rate of acquisitions, and careful planning of new academic programs. These strategies were to become all too familiar and were unable to provide the magic bullet to library cost containment. It is important in reviewing Cummings's remarks to note that he was writing in a pre-Internet world, one which did not offer the range of alternative solutions to the crisis in journal pricing that are today available. However, it is equally important to note that even from today's perspective, librarians are still discussing these economic issues and alternative solutions without genuine resolution to the problems they are facing. Cummings's work gave the necessary stimulus to the Association of Research Libraries to maintain its much-cited annual studies of the growth curves in the purchase of library materials, and the annual costs. These studies begin with base year 1986 and are published annually in the introduction to the annual compilations of research library statistics. The value is, of course, in the accumulation of uniform data over time. The 2004 edition of this annual statistical compilation notes that "library material budgets have risen sharply in order to sustain serial expenditures."[9] We will return to these annual statistics in our discussion on the Big Deal later in this chapter.

Medical librarians have enjoyed for decades the benefit of a carefully controlled longitudinal study of the costs of medical books and periodicals, the familiar "Brandon/Hill list," as it is affectionately known by its eponym. This selected list of books and journals for the medical library began in 1965 and appeared annually in the *Journal of the Medical Library Association.* It uses a different approach from the ARL data since it looks at the prices of particular publications and tracks their cost increases over time; it does not review acquisition rates in libraries. This list, with its systematic study of the cost of library materials in relation to the U.S. Consumer Price Index, is an invaluable objective tool used by medical librarians around the world. Its unbiased findings concluded in 2004:

> The result of the 2002 update shows that the average price continues to be independent of the low inflation rate in evidence for over a decade. The authors find that prices have jumped 51.90% from 1996 to 1999 and 32% from 1999 to 2002 which is consistent with nearly every recent study of journal prices. *Library Journal* reports a 35.63% price increase for health sciences journals from 1999 to 2003 while the American Library Association's *U.S. Periodical Price Index* of 2002 shows increases of 53.20% from 1996 to 1999 and 29.30% from 1999 to 2002 for journals in medicine. The most recent *Index Medicus* price study indicates an average price increase of 51.50% for the period 1994 to 1998 with 32% of these titles showing an increase of 200% or higher.[10]

Having documented the continuing and high rate of increase on the study group of medical journals, the authors conclude that the significant and unprecedented cost increases have had a strong negative impact on the ability of medical librarians to provide access to necessary information. This was a clarion call to the community of librarians who held, as a core value over its history, the provision of access to information. Solutions had to be found, ones that included aggressive fund-raising both within and outside the librarian's institution, the evolution of cooperative acquisition of electronic resources within library consortia, and the purchase of an entire publishers' output at a reduced cost per title.

THE SEARCH FOR NEW SOLUTIONS: THE "BIG DEAL"

More fundamental than the economics of the journal publishing industry was the change in scientific communication and publishing brought about by the digital revolution. The digital and information revolution provided new business opportunities, and more important, it created new ways of doing business that raised the question of who really owned the "business." Change in scientific publishing had begun decades earlier with the preparation and submission of journal articles in digital form. With the Internet, the entire production system could "go" digital and the end of the printed journal was a matter of time. Improved turnaround time in publishing and great improvements in ease and speed of access to readers proved a compelling inducement to the users of the scientific and medical literature to move toward the digital library. Initial concerns were expressed by librarians regarding the permanence of digital archives, but in the hierarchy of librarians' values, the question of access took precedence over the question of permanence. Besides, there was considerable effort being undertaken, in very large medical libraries and elsewhere, to guarantee the perpetuation of the digital archive.

A number of alternatives began to be explored as the result of these changes. In the library community, intensified library collaboration through collective purchasing of packages of electronic journals emerged as the dominant response. In the research and scholarly communities, some of the new initiatives, BioMed Central, BioOne, and The Public Library of Science, among others, presented a much greater potential challenge to the dominant commercial publishing model. These are explored in chapter 10 on open access. Although important in their potential, the entire "market share" of these publishing alternatives is less than 5 percent of global publishing in science, technical, and medical information. For the moment, librarians are not able to turn to these alternatives to solve their economic woes, since most of the titles to which they need to provide access are published by mainstream commercial publishers. The ecology of scholarly communication and the public purse will determine the final outcome.

The benefits of electronic journals were undeniable. But for librarians and their administrators they were to prove a mixed blessing, in large measure because of the costs of these publications and the introduction of the concept of the "Big Deal." The Big Deal has been defined as "any online aggregation of e-content that a publisher, aggregator or vendor offers for sale or lease at prices and/or terms that substantially encourages acquisition of the entire corpus."[11] By the mid-1990s librarians had diligently added to their list of requisite skills the mastering of legal licensing agreements to provide limited user access to the full package of journals made available by a particular publisher using the concept of the Big Deal. These were essential survival skills, and they were accompanied by the librarian's recognition of the fundamental change in the relationship between the library and the information the library was acquiring in digital form. No longer was an item of information owned in perpetuity, as in the case of the purchase of a printed book, for example. Even if librarians canceled subscriptions to printed journals, the retrospective issues of the title still resided on the library shelves. They had been bought and were the property of the library. In the digital world, what is being purchased is not a copy of the journal but the right to access the information contained in it during the time period covered by the license. The shift from ownership to access was accompanied by changes in what the licensee was allowed to do with the licensed information. To protect their ownership rights and to maximize revenue streams, electronic journal publishers placed limitations on what the librarian was permitted to do, especially in the areas of interlibrary loan and document delivery. Librarians found themselves making photocopies of electronic journal articles and faxing these to a user on interlibrary loan, rather than simply forwarding an electronic copy of the article, since such forwarding to a nonmember of the licensed organization was forbidden. The old concept of fair use was being eliminated by the conditions of the contract that the librarian had signed with the publishers. These restrictions struck at the ability of the librarian to deliver information wherever it is needed, a core value of the profession. Discussion with publishers at meetings of professional librarians continues to be characterized by a proactive approach to resolving these issues. Contract law, as exemplified in licensing agreements, seemed to be replacing the fundamental common law (and common sense!) concept of "fair use" as it is known in the United States or "fair dealing" in Canada.

As librarians developed their skills in negotiating site licenses and their understanding of contract law in the process of making the best possible arrangements with publishers, they shared their experiences. Certain guiding principles or, more practically put, "show stoppers," became part of a collective response from the librarian community in all its specialties, in determining whether a license allowed the librarian the right to perform essential duties. Most important from the perspective of the medical and hospital librarian was the inclusion of an appropriate and comprehensive definition of the primary user group, those entitled to access the information by virtue of their membership in the institution regardless of their location. This has proven to be one of the more difficult issues in health information delivery involving commercial databases. Other key issues that concerned librarians were transparency in the pricing of the product and continuing access to the archive of the publisher if a license is cancelled. At an early stage in the development of consortia for licensing electronic information, useful advice began to appear in medical and university library literature regarding the negotiation of site licenses.[12]

Licensing skills are a growth area in librarianship. As consortia proliferate, much of the licensing for a group of libraries is typically delegated to a single individual, either to a permanent staff member of the consortium office, in the case of a consortium large enough to afford a permanent secretariat, or to a staff member in one of the member libraries who has proven ability in this area. But although responsibility may be delegated outside of the organization, librarians have found that they must stay on top of the detail. The parent institution of the library often become involved as well, especially in the case of large financial commitments, and some institutions require a reading of the license by the legal counsel of the university. It seems at times that the individual user of the library around whose needs these services are being built is increasingly remote from this process. The librarian may be frustrated by the complexities involved in providing the mere opportunity to the users of the library to read a given article. In consulting the online catalog, the librarian and the user alike may be astonished to learn that the library has licensed multiple copies of the same electronic journal. Packaging and repackaging of specialized information make the unraveling of duplication an unsolved problem in today's electronic library.

Today, packages or bundles of electronic journals are the standard method for acquiring access to the medical and scientific journal literature. Much is at stake here for librarians in supporting access to information, and one dominant strategy that has engaged most academic libraries by the late 1990s was consortial purchasing. Library consortia and collectives already existed for decades, and these provided a logical forum for the negotiation of collective purchasing agreements. Where they did not exist, consortia could be easily invented as a means of securing purported reductions in costs through collective agreements involving multiple libraries. In retrospect, these arrangements are likely to be viewed, at their best, as mid-term tactics in the "publishers wars," a limited success in providing improved access but at a very high cost, with respect both to price and to control of the budget and collection.

Cooperation is deeply embedded in the practice of medical librarianship, and it may appear counterproductive to question the value of consortium activity at the time of great opportunity. It is important to clarify that it is not cooperation or consortium participation per se that is being questioned; it is the particular negotiation of large-scale multi-institutional arrangements between a group of libraries and a particular publisher that requires revisiting. Much has been written on this topic—on the subject of reduced costs, the provision of access to more titles by more users at the same cost, and the predictability of multiyear budgets given the pricing structure. The strongest argument in favor of the Big Deal is probably that more researchers get access to more materials even if they are at smaller institutions. This is commonly referred to as "leveling the playing field."

One aspect of the use of the Big Deal that proved particularly challenging, after the question of costs, was the loss of control of the collection in the face of an all-or-none approach to a publisher's entire output. This loss was experienced at various levels: at the interuniversity level there was a loss of independent decision making because the library of a particular institution was one of a number of participating institutions. Within an institution, decisions were being made on behalf of all disciplines, with medicine only one of the many disciplines to be considered in the journal "package." This was not problematic for several reasons, not the least of which was the well-developed communication between the medical library and other campus libraries. More important intellectually was the overlap between medical science and other sciences and the ease of access to publications that were of relevance to a number of different user communities. However, a more serious issue was the threat to the well-established relationship in the network that consisted of the academic medical library and the libraries located in the various local hospitals. Resource sharing in this network had traditionally built upon a complex set of cross-appointments between the university, the medical school, and the hospital, and the relationship between teaching, research, and clinical practice. But the licensing agreements often separated the university from the hospital and threatened to create a barrier to access. Solutions with varying degrees of effectiveness were developed. Of course, it was always possible to pay more or to create separate licensing agreements. Another solution was for vendors to acknowledge that staff were jointly appointed to the university and the hospital. This solved the problem for clinical practitioners who held joint appointments but not for other staff in the hospitals. Walk-in use, defined as use by anyone who walks into the library, was soon permitted by many publishers, but this again was only partially effective since it failed to allow direct access on wards, the nursing station, or any place outside the medical library, which is where the medical literature was likely to be of use.

The Big Deal rapidly became the dominant method of providing access to the journal literature in medicine and science. Several factors contributed to its rapid adoption. It has helped libraries move more quickly into the electronic era by a pricing structure that came to encourage the cancellation of print subscriptions and the reliance upon electronic versions of journal articles. Another reason has been the acquisition of additional funding, usually from the government, to provide for collective consortial participation at a regional or national level.

THE CANADIAN "REALLY BIG" DEAL

The Canadian experience can serve as a useful example of effective fund development to promote the Big Deal at a national level. Like librarians in many countries, Canadian librarians had banded together in the print era to obtain price reductions on publications and to rationalize the purchase of costly publications through resource sharing. Collaboration became more intense in the 1980s as the ability of librarians to provide users with the necessary information was in jeopardy due to increasing cost escalation, as discussed earlier. The need for resource-sharing agreements that optimized the institution's investment was clear. In Canada, four strong regional consortia had developed that connected research libraries, including the nation's sixteen medical school libraries from Newfoundland in the east to Vancouver Island in the west. These consortia, from west to east, are

- the prairies and the west—The Council of Prairies and Pacific University Libraries (COPPUL), consisting of Canada's western provinces: British Columbia, Alberta, Saskatchewan, and Manitoba
- the province of Ontario—The Ontario Council of University Libraries (OCUL)
- the province of Québec—Conference des recteurs et principaux des universités du Quebéc (CREPUQ) Sous-comité des bibliothèques
- the Atlantic provinces, including New Brunswick, Nova Scotia, Prince Edward Island, and Newfoundland: The Council of Atlantic University Libraries (CAUL)

In 1997, the Canadian federal government announced the creation of the Canadian Foundation for Innovation (CFI). This program was designed to invest in the nation's research infrastructure. It would provide the Canadian medical, scientific, and research communities with the necessary tools to conduct high-level research and stimulate creativity in the sciences. Funding under the CFI would be provided to a maximum of 40 percent of the capital costs. Part of the additional money required (40 percent) was to come from the ten provincial governments of Canada in support of successful CFI applications, thereby maintaining the delicate balance of power that exists between Canada's federal and provincial governments. The final 20 percent was to be provided from other partners, including the institutional recipients. This program has been enormously successful and has been renewed twice since its beginning. The Canadian library community continues its involvement in the program. However, it is the initial experience with the first grants to libraries that is of special relevance to our discussion. It also must be emphasized that while the initiative of a national consortium was a unique and a "Very Big Deal" for Canada, for purposes of comparison, the investment is roughly equal in size to that of the state of California.

Libraries were not considered eligible initially for participation under the CFI granting initiative, as they were not considered to be part of the research and innovation community. Intense and prolonged discussions had to take place between CFI program officers and librarians, at both the regional and national level, to create the necessary conditions for the acceptance of a proposal from the library community. The Canadian Association of Research Libraries (CARL), consisting of the heads of the twenty-eight major research libraries from across Canada, was to play a major role in transforming this situation to the benefit of libraries. The most compelling argument put forward from this group was that the information provided to the medical and research communities by libraries was essential to the research that was being conducted. Scientific research would suffer, it was argued, if an appropriate information infrastructure, analogous to computer infrastructure, was not available to the community of researchers. The conclusion was indeed most beneficial for libraries because it was finally agreed that an information infrastructure was essential to the development of research. With this revised clarification in hand, librarians from each of Canada's four major consortia prepared proposals, with the essential component in each proposal being a list of electronic journal packages from large publishers. When these four proposals were reviewed, this similarity was not lost upon the referees for the CFI. The granting agency advised that what they wished to see from the librarians was an integration of these regional proposals into a single national site-licensing initiative. In the summer of 1999, CFI announced a grant of $20 million to support the Canadian National Site Licensing Project (CNSLP). By now, membership in the consortium had been enlarged to include sixty-four Canadian libraries providing support to the Canadian research community. This enlargement of participation is important because it emphasizes strong support for making research information available to all who need to use it, the core value of librarians. The proposal's strength lay in the fact that it provided the same level of access to quality scientific and medical information to someone in a remote and small institution as that available to a researcher at a large, research-intensive university.

The national experiment with CFI/CNSLP can provide a useful perspective for evaluating the consortium experiment as a means for providing enhanced access to packages of electronic information. At the outset, this grant was given over a finite three-year period; as a demonstration project, an exit strategy was essential. But in point of fact, there could be no real exit from the provision of essential medical and scientific information. What was accomplished was the clear acceptance of the fact that researchers wanted and needed enhanced access to electronic information and there was no going back on this commitment. After the three years of the CFI national grant, universities struggled to provide their libraries with the funds to absorb the costs that the grant had temporarily eliminated or drastically reduced. The bottom line was that the dominant model that had emerged in large universities for the delivery of medical and scientific information—the purchase of bundled subscriptions from large commercial publishers—had been reinforced and extended by the CNSLP experience.[13]

The Canadian experience in national consortial activity was highly successful as a temporary strategy. Canadian librarians enthusiastically supported the initiative from its inception, although medical librarians were vigilant to ensure that the needs of their particular users were being met. And there would always be certain databases that were of interest only to the medical community. The experiment had provided new resources for a limited period and, most important, had advanced the use of electronic information. It had made scientific and medical information resources available to a larger community, as the national site licenses included users at many smaller institutions outside the major urban centers.

QUESTIONING THE BIG DEAL

The university research library community was alert to the implications of the Big Deal. In explaining certain trends in research library statistics in 2003, the annual ARL survey notes that

> During the past five years, libraries have expanded the amount of material to which they provide access by purchasing the same content in new formats and acquiring new content, often through bundling arrangements as well as by managing the growing amount of content available through the open-access mechanisms. The purchase of new and dual-format content via bundling or "big deal" arrangements is probably partly responsible for the recent decline in the growth rate for serial unit costs—libraries have added serial titles to their collections at lower incremental prices. These additional titles are often duplicate subscriptions or titles the library would not otherwise purchase. Depending on the publishers' financial model some of the additional content may be purchased or some may come bundled or "free" with a subscription to other products.[14]

This explanation reveals the dilemma in which the library community was being placed. Titles were being purchased in duplicate, titles that were not completely necessary, it would seem, and yet unit costs per title were declining. However, overall subscription costs were increasing. As the millennium turned, some librarians were reacting to the dominant purchasing paradigm inherent in the Big Deal, based on leadership within the library community.[15]

University librarians and others representing major research institutions in the United States—Cornell University, Harvard University, and the Libraries of the University of California system—had begun to revolt under the economic yoke of the Big Deal. The University of California insisted on a license to selected titles only, rather than the comprehensive package of journals provided under Elsevier's Science Direct collective package of journal titles. Daniel Greenstein spoke out on the need for action and for new alternatives to the Big Deal:

> I believe that the business model of commercial publishing which once served the academy's information needs now threatens fundamentally to undermine and pervert the course of research and teaching. Put bluntly, the model is economically unsustainable for us. If business as usual continues, it will deny scholars both access to the information they need and the ability to distribute their work to the worldwide audience it deserves.[16]

Using information obtained from Bear Stearns Investment Bank, Greenstein notes increases in subscription prices from 1986 to 2002 that were four times higher than the consumer price index rate of inflation. Costs of annual subscriptions rose 227 percent over the sixteen-year period, but the consumer price index a mere 57 percent. During the period covered by the figures quoted by Greenstein, librarians increasingly had employed the strategy of the Big Deal as a perceived economy of the "more for less" variety. However, by the end of the century the economic catastrophe of very high and ever increasing costs and the limited budgets of libraries had reached a watershed.

Librarians attempted to use a time-honored strategy of "scaling down" to address the shortfalls in their budgets and the escalating costs of bundled journal subscriptions. However, when they applied the familiar practice of canceling individual journal titles within the context of bundled subscriptions, retaining only those titles that they needed, they soon found that pricing for selective titles was discriminatory, providing fewer titles at a far greater unit cost per title. Some librarians, working closely with academic administrators and faculty, persevered, believing that these cost increases per individual title were the price that had to be paid if librarians were to repatriate control over their collections—a worthy intellectual argument but not likely to resonate in the accounting department of a university. Most librarians continue to place high value on providing access to the largest number of titles, and publishers renegotiate their initial price in order to maintain the present practice. At times, librarians appear united with large commercial publishers to save the phenomenon.

Discussions of the Big Deal have proliferated on university campuses, and some faculties are becoming actively engaged in the issues of journal costs and reform of the system of scholarly communication. One faculty member, a chemist from the University of California, noted that commercial publishers received an increasingly large share of the serial budget of the library at the University: "Elsevier has raked in 50 percent of the online journal budget for 32 percent of the titles and only 25 percent of the use. In my discipline, chemistry, rather few of these titles are amongst the best. Journals from professional societies are typically much cheaper and of better quality."[17]

The question of whether it is possible for a library consortium to withdraw from the Big Deal and continue to act in the public interest of users has been raised in OhioLINK. This statewide consortium, one of the most successful consortia with eighty-five institutional members, is well known through the speaking and writing of Tom Sanville, director of OhioLINK, for its careful statistical methods in documenting and analyzing user behavior.[18] The lessons of the OhioLINK consortium inform the reasoning that the selection of individual titles as opposed to the licensing of the comprehensive list of a publisher's output has a net result of users placing limits on access to information. OhioLINK statistics have shown that if the information is there, it will be used: titles that became available following the implementation of a Big Deal that were previously not held by any member of the consortium were actively used once they became available. Different member institutions use different titles, and the strategy of canceling selected titles is no longer viable in a consortium setting. At the heart of the argument is a support of the Big Deal, a concept worth saving. According to Gatten and Sanville, it is "deemed a reasonable and cost effective approach to expanding access to scholarly information because it demonstrates that title-by-title collection development selections do not adequately address user needs."[19] The answer lies in a negotiated agreement with publishers for "incremental attrition." One need not reason too closely to understand the long-term implications of the strategy of incremental attrition. Data from the OhioLINK consortium demonstrated that a minority of titles (approximately 30 percent) accounted for a majority (more than

80 percent of the articles downloaded from any one publisher). The question that librarians were beginning to ask was whether all those less-used titles were sufficiently valued to justify the cost.

Librarians from all specialties in the profession have common cause in negotiating access to the journal literature; medical, science, university, and hospital librarians alike are impacted by the high and increasing costs of providing access to the journal literature. The costs of these licenses, high at the point of initial signing, become an even greater challenge at the time of renewal. Publishers use a variety of strategies, sometimes negotiating with individual libraries at a preferred rate for participation and challenging others to participate or experience the criticism of users for failing to subscribe. The threat of charging based upon cost per use intimidates some libraries because of their higher use and the uncontrollable costs that result from being unable to predict what a user may need. Librarians have intensified their collaborative discussions. They are becoming more aggressive in engaging their campus or hospital administration regarding the economics of information. These discussions often prove most informative and positive since senior administrators often have only a vague idea of the costs of journals. Users became part of the strategy, and a specific target group was members of the editorial boards of journals. These faculty were normally donating their services to publishers during the editorial process while those same publishers were extracting increasingly high costs from the institutions through the costs that libraries were incurring in purchasing the same journals in which they were publishing their research. The dilemma for all librarians was the perception held by publishers and, surprisingly, by a few librarians themselves that the crisis was not in the pricing of journals but in library funding; simply put, if only institutions provided their libraries with more money there would be no problem.

Most librarians were not susceptible to the explanation that the crisis was simply one of library funding, since they had seen the disproportionate reallocation of library budgets at an institutional level to accommodate the high cost of medical and scientific journals. Harvard University was one of a number of major universities in the United States, including the libraries of the University of California system, Cornell, and the University of North Carolina, that moved to curb the unbridled expansion of the Big Deal. After more than one year of deliberations, Sidney Verba, Carl H. Pforzheimer University professor and director of the university library at Harvard, announced cancellation of the Big Deal and noted that this decision "was driven not only by current financial realities, but also, and perhaps more importantly, by the need to reassert control over our collection and to encourage new models for research publication at Harvard."[20] Harvard had reacted to the bundling of journal subscriptions that compelled libraries to allocate a large fixed amount of the budget to a publisher, regardless of whether all the titles were relevant and important to campus users of the library. They had decided to purchase online access to journals on a title-by-title basis rather than to contract for a global license that would have increased by $500,000 in five years.

At Cornell University, the library, under the leadership of Sarah Thomas, launched a public-awareness campaign among users and administrators against the high costs of commercial publishers and the bundling of journal subscriptions. Librarians were willing to pay the twofold costs of losing access to some less-used titles and of an increasing cost per title received in order to assert their unique campus needs and to reject the bundled package offered by Elsevier.[21] Similar educational efforts and support from users occurred on the Stanford University campus. In early 2004, the Faculty Senate of the University endorsed a motion that the libraries "cancel some costly journal subscriptions and faculty withhold articles and reviews from publishers who engage in questionable pricing practices. The motion singled out publishing giant Elsevier as deserving special attention."[22] Michael Keller, chief librarian, describes the fundamental reason for these actions. Keller emphasized that this was not a short-term tactic to better position his institution in negotiating price with commercial publishers. The motivation was far more revolutionary: to push forward a new system of scholarly communication in the journal literature. Stanford libraries were not reacting to the Big Deal per se, since at the time they did not have one. They subscribed to only 400 carefully selected titles from Elsevier, well less than half of the Elsevier titles published. In 2004, these 400 titles cost them slightly less than one million dollars. The library spent some six million dollars on 23,000 titles annually. Put another way, approximately 20 percent of the annual budget was spent on acquiring between 1 and 2 percent of the titles represented by Elsevier publications in the Stanford collections. At Stanford's Lane Medical Library, with its separate administrative structure, the ratios were verified to be approximately the same.

Saying "no" to the Big Deal is not an easy or a frequent choice for most librarians. Rather, the continued financial support of their institutions and other funding sources keeps the process in place. In fairness, many are caught in the dilemma of not wanting to take a position that may appear confrontational or, even worse, place the primary objective of the library, providing information services, in jeopardy. Wishing to encourage use and expand service, they may look for alternatives. One such approach is being explored in Great Britain. Librarians there recognized clearly that many of the titles received in the comprehensive packages of journals licensed from publishers were not necessarily those most wanted by their particular users. Further, because of the high and ever increasing cost of these bundled journals, cuts were occurring in other parts of the collections in order to meet these costs. There was less control over information resources development in the best interests of a particular user group. Journals less needed within an institution had to be retained if they were part of the package, and other titles that might be more relevant were being cancelled to release funds for the large packages. As a result, librarians in Britain are exploring the possibility of a "core plus peripheral" approach.[23] As the name suggests, institutions would purchase sets of titles from a publisher in a particular discipline. Access to articles in journals not included in this more precisely defined set of core titles would then be available on a pay-per-view basis. The pros and cons of this model are being carefully evaluated in an effort that seems determined to "preserve the phenomena" with the least disruption to the status quo.

Despite the growing dissatisfaction with the present economic model of delivering bundled journal subscriptions to libraries, there appears to be reluctance on the part of librarians, with some significant exceptions, to abandon the ease and reliability of the present system. Alternatives promise dramatic reductions in subscription costs when fully developed, but many of these are not fully in place, nor has the durability of their business models been tested. These alternatives represent a truly radical rethinking of the present system of scholarly communication—a paradigm shift in the most legitimate sense of the term. We shall examine these alternatives and their growth in the following chapters.

NOTES

1. Peter Stangl [letter to the editor], *Bulletin of the Medical Library Association* 77, no. 1 (January 1989): 80–84.

2. Stangl [letter to the editor], 81.

3. Alan R. Liss [letter to the editor], *Bulletin of the Medical Library Association* 77, no. 1 (January 1989): 84 (italics added).

4. Gary D. Byrd, "An Economic Commons' Tragedy for Research Libraries: Scholarly Journal Publishing and Pricing Trends," *College and Research Libraries* 51, no. 3 (1990): 184–95.

5. Lelde B. Gilman, "The Scholarly Publishing Imbroglio: A Personal View," *Bulletin of the Medical Library Association* 79, no. 1 (January 1991): 88–92.

6. Gilman, "The Scholarly Publishing Imbroglio," 89.

7. Joint Funding Council's Libraries Review Group, Report (The Follett Report) December, 1993 (Report for Higher Education Funding, Council for England, Scottish Higher Education Funding Council, Higher Education Funding Council for Wales, and Department of Education for Northern Ireland), http://www.ukoln.ac.uk/services/papers/follett/report/ (accessed March 23, 2006).

8. Martin M. Cummings, *The Economics of Research Libraries*. (Washington, DC: Council on Library Resources, 1986), 146.

9. Martha Kyrillidou and Mark Young, eds., *ARL Statistics, 2002–2003: A Compilation of Statistics from One Hundred and Twenty-three Members of the Association of Research Libraries* (Washington, DC: Association of Research Libraries, 2004).

10. Joan B. Schlimgren and Michael R. Kronenfeld, "Update on Inflation of Journal Prices: Brandon/Hill List Journals and the Scientific, Technical and Medical Publishing Market," *Journal of the Medical Library Association* 92, no. 3 (July 2004): 307.

11. Thomas A. Peters, "What's a Big Deal?" *Journal of Academic Librarianship* 27, no. 4 (July 2001): 302–4.

12. One noteworthy example of the guidance that appeared at an earlier stage is Ann Okerson, "What Academic Libraries Need in Electronic Content Licenses: Presentation to the STM Library Relations Committee, STM Annual General Meeting, October 1, 1996," *Serials Review* 22, no. 4 (Winter, 1996): 65–72.

13. Frances Groen, "Canada's National Initiative to Advance Access to Electronic Journals," *Health Libraries Review* 17, no. 4 (December 2000): 189–93.

14. Kyrillidou and Young, eds., *ARL Statistics, 2002–2003*.

15. See especially the work of Kenneth Frazier, for example, "The Librarians' Dilemma: Contemplating the Costs of the 'Big Deal,'" *D-Lib Magazine* 7, no. 3 (March 2001).

16. Daniel Greenstein, "Not So Quiet on the Western Front," http://www.nature.com/nature/focus/accessdebate/23.html (accessed November 17, 2004).

17. A. Christopher, "Just Say No to Exploitative Publishers of Science Journals," *Chronicle of Higher Education*, February 24, 2004, http://reedgroup.ucr.edu/justsaynotoexploitativepublishersofsciencejournals.htm (accessed November 17, 2004).

18. Jeffrey N. Gatten and Tom Sanville, "An Orderly Retreat from the Big Deal: Is It Possible for Consortia?" *D-Lib Magazine* no. 10 (2004), http://www.dlib.org/dlib/october04/gatten/10gatten.html (accessed October 15, 2004).

19. Gatten and Sanville, "An Orderly Retreat from the Big Deal."

20. *Harvard University Gazette*, February 5, 2004, http://www/news.harvard.edu/gazette/2004/02.05/10-libraries.html (accessed November 17, 2004).

21. "Cornell Axes Elsevier Journals as Prices Rise," *Nature* 426 (November 20, 2003): 217.

22. Ray Delgado, "Faculty Senate Approves Resolution Regarding Pricey Journals, Stanford Librarian Hopes the Move Will Convince Other Universities to Can-

cel Subscriptions, Leading to Industry Reforms," *Stanford Report*, February 25, 2004, http://news-service.stanford.edu/news/2004/february25/journals-225.html (accessed November 27, 2004).

23. Hugh Look, "The UK Perspective: The JISC Business Models Report," (presentation at the JISC International Colloquium, London, June 22, 2005), http:www.jisc.ac.uk/uploaded_documents/Hugh%20Look.ppt (accessed March 19, 2006).

10

TOWARD OPEN ACCESS

A PRELUDE TO OPEN ACCESS

The development of the open-access movement is deeply rooted in the history of scientific communication in the form of the scientific journal, referred to here as scientific journalism. Quantitative studies of the growth and structure of scientific literature have emerged in the last thirty years in the wake of the pioneering work of Derek de Solla Price.[1] The concepts of the "gift culture" and the "Matthew effect" that reinforce the existing rewards system in the sense that "unto him who hath is given" have been studied by sociologists, in particular by Robert K. Merton and his disciples[2] and have become part of our understanding of scientific communication. In 1979, William Garvey adopted a different approach from these earlier studies in *Communication: The Essence of Science*,[3] which examined the work habits of practicing scientists. Garvey wanted to uncover how scientific researchers behaved, and his study concentrated on concrete issues—for example, the proportion of research time spent on communication. Garvey's volume also dealt with pragmatic questions of improving the concrete processes of scientific communication. Although Garvey's pragmatic approach was aimed primarily at solving some practical managerial questions, it nonetheless managed to address some fundamental questions relating to the nature of science. For scientists, communication does not simply mean transferring knowledge results from individual to individual; it also contributes to the structuring of scientific communities, including their inherent pecking order and their power structure. Evaluating, reviewing, and gatekeeping are activities practiced in the name of excellence, but they also reflect various hierarchies among researchers and even contribute to reinforcing them. Neglecting these issues could only limit and ultimately distort our vision of science.

The emergence of electronic publishing fueled the revisiting of the study of scientific communication because publishing, as part of scientific communication, was at the very heart of the practice of science. Many of the issues tied to the print culture had become so deeply embedded within a familiar landscape that they had essentially become invisible. But the emergence of electronic publishing in scientific communication brought many of these issues to the surface, and as a result, scholars and historians are revisiting the "Gutenberg galaxy," to use Marshall McLuhan's famous phrase. In the process, not only has new territory been uncovered, but issues of control and power have also taken center stage. In parallel, these new studies have tended to demonstrate how human relationships, text-human symbiosis, and intertext weaving have been deeply affected and reorganized by the advent of the revolution in scientific communication in the Internet era.

The presence of a multiplicity of favorable, but disconnected, elements alone could not have accounted for the development of an open-access movement. More direct factors had to be in place before open access could even be imagined. Chapter 6 describes the creation of the revolution in communications technology that transformed the library world and provided a necessary condition for the development of open access. Necessary, but not sufficient: it was also necessary to move beyond technology and consider issues of the right to access information in the public good, the mentality of sharing and exchanging scientific information, and the history and economics of scientific and medical publishing.

During the Depression years with the concomitant decreases in library budgets, librarians felt the need at an early stage to use scarce financial resources as effectively as possible. To assist them in purchasing only the most important works from their limited budgets, a number of statistical analyses of book usage within libraries were undertaken. Best known and still quoted today is the work of Samuel Clemens Bradford, a British librarian whose work was built upon the recognition that the ratio of cost to use was the crucial parameter. In 1934 Bradford enunciated a distribution law that that came to be known as Bradford's law, or Bradford's law of scatter, which asserts that the most significant articles in any given field of investigation are found within a relatively small group of publications.[4] Bradford showed that to make a number of useful references grow arithmetically, one needed to canvas a number of titles that grew at a geometric rate.[5] The consequence of this law was that libraries increasingly organized their collections according to the needs of their constituencies, which was to be expected. In doing so, librarians were now empowered with a precise mathematical tool that helped calculate what was really useful. However, the unintended consequence of the application of Bradford's law was that, given the ways in which one university faculty resembles another in terms of the research agenda, skills, and needs, a gradual convergence of purchasing profiles began to emerge. Libraries began to purchase journals in an increasingly precise fashion, eliminating less-used titles. As a consequence, library collections came to resemble each other to an ever increasing degree.

The combination of returning U.S. servicemen who took advantage of the postwar GI Bill that provided free college education and the realization of the importance of defense technology swelled the ranks of scientists and scientific publications. Two problems emerged from this new situation. On the one hand, it was necessary to accommodate all these new papers—an objective that could be reached by increasing the size of individual journals and multiplying titles. In the latter case, this opened up new opportunities for commercial publishers, as they could offer their services more quickly than learned societies or scientific associations. The second problem was related to the tracking of this flood of literature. Bibliographies began losing ground, and a debate began emerging in the 1950s about science drowning in its own information because the bibliographies were coming in too slowly, condemning many researchers to revisit problems already satisfactorily treated elsewhere. As the number of productive (i.e., publishing) scientists grew, so did the number of papers, and problems of information control, access, and dissemination, always a concern for medical librarians, were becoming acute. The rapid growth of literature also led to a more rapid evolution of scientific domains and the emergence of a number of new interdisciplinary fields that were difficult to cover because, by definition, they tended to straddle various disciplines and, therefore, bibliographies. Molecular biology—a domain that was exploding by the 1960s—provides a good example of this kind of difficulty. One of its most prominent practitioners bears an already familiar name: the Nobel Prize winner, Joshua Lederberg.

The bibliographic crisis coupled with the surge of interdisciplinary fields of research that were poorly covered by traditional bibliographic tools stimulated inventiveness. Its most lasting and well-known result was the *Science Citation Index (SCI)*, designed by Eugene Garfield. Garfield's brilliant concept consisted in following up the paper trail of citations across scientific articles. This concept was rooted in the work done by American lawyer Frank Shepard in the later part of the nineteenth century that had produced a citation index for case law: a lawyer located a case similar to one he was working on and consulted Shepard's Citator to determine whether later cases had cited it.[6] What is not so well known or understood is how Garfield managed to make this concept operational. Clearly, tracing all the citations of all the articles in all scientific articles of the world was not humanly possible and was also beyond the capability of even the most powerful computers at the beginning of the 1960s. Further, even if the possibility existed, the results would be unmanageable. However, cutting the problem down to size threatened to give a false idea of the scientific trail of citations. For this reason, Garfield had to find a way to justify his drastic simplification of the world's scientific publishing system. To do so, he constructed an argument based on Bradford's law of distribution, but taking it backward. Rather than paying attention to the indefinite extension of research to obtain the ideal, total, exhaustive bibliography, he decided to look at what was needed to reach an acceptable result. His reasoning is based on what is commonly referred to as the Pareto principle, which asserts that 80 percent of use or need is met by 20 percent of the available resources. Conversely, an additional 80 percent of resources is needed to satisfy the remaining 20 percent of needs. Garfield made some calculations to imagine how many titles he needed to canvas to be able to survey a significant fraction of the citations to ensure a result that could be both credible and useful. His initial estimates led him to a figure lower than one thousand titles. This became his starting point for the *Science Citation Index*. It also led to defining a set of journals that quickly drifted over to becoming a "core set" of journal titles, and this core set, in turn, quickly evolved to equate to something entirely new and with deep implications—namely "core science." From now on, there would be two kinds of science: core science and all the rest, left unnamed by Garfield, but regarded as peripheral or marginal science.

During the same period that Eugene Garfield was developing his *SCI*, the commercial publishing sector was active in improving its understanding of the financial benefits of acquiring ownership of scientific journals. Subsequently, the merger of publishing firms and association publishers became an important strategic advantage. The business of commercial journal publishing became big business indeed. One particular history, that of Pergamon Press and its founder, Robert Maxwell, illustrates these dynamics. It is quite probable that no one saw the commercial potential of science publishing as clearly as Robert Maxwell. Maxwell, born Jan Luvik Huk, escaped Nazi persecution of the Jews in his native Czechoslovakia by fleeing to England in 1940. Immediately after the war, he began to advance in the Allied Control Commission in Berlin. In 1951, he bought for thirteen thousand pounds a company called Pergamon, which had originally been set up by Butterworth and Springer to import Springer Verlag books into

Britain. In terms of publishing, Pergamon in 1951 dealt with only six titles. As Brian Cox, a longtime employee of Pergamon, recounts, "The secret of Pergamon was the scientific journal. Most new Pergamon journal titles started with the same three words: *International Journal of. . . .*"[7]

Robert Maxwell and Eugene Garfield met in the late 1950s, well before the success or even the beginning of *SCI*, and it is clear that Maxwell, intent as he obviously was to create a space for commercial publishing in science,[8] had quickly grasped the possibilities of *SCI*. As Eugene Garfield recounts:

> Over the next 35 years he tried to acquire my company in one way or another. I've briefly described our relations in the oral interview recently recorded by Bob Williams. One day I will describe in detail about how he tried but failed. He was a diabolical, driven genius. Fortunately, the competitive world of publishing is full of people who live and let live.[9]

What ways Maxwell used to try to acquire *SCI* remain unsaid, but the characterization of "a diabolical, driven genius" leaves little doubt as to the probable ferocity of the confrontation between Maxwell and Garfield.

What the presence and activities of Robert Maxwell actually signal is a phenomenon that has been discussed very little, although it is undoubtedly of great importance: the transformations of science after WWII essentially led to a very profound change in the system of scientific communication. The most important result of this change was the emergence of a dynamic, profit-driven publishing sector in an area that hitherto had been dominated by "genteel" society publishers, to use Brian Cox's word. It might not be out of place to call it a revolution, except for the fact that most revolutionary periods are not as quiet or invisible as this particular one. But, as we shall see, scholarly publishing has been revolutionized, not once, not twice, but at least four times between the 1950s and the Budapest Open Access Initiative in 2002.

The reason Robert Maxwell eyed *SCI* with such intensity is easy to imagine. *SCI* reinforced the inelastic market that Bradford's law had already, albeit unwittingly, helped to found, and Maxwell obviously fully understood the financial implications of that fact. But one may imagine what would have happened if Maxwell had also had the tools to shape the contours of that inelastic market. He would likely have created many more journals than he did. Moreover, he could have promoted all or at least most of them almost at will. With the transformations experienced by the science publishing market, this line of business had already moved to the level of a respectable money pump.

Had Maxwell succeeded, he would have been able to take a commanding position within the science publishing system of the world.

The success of Pergamon was based on an exponential growth in science journal publishing, especially in an international content. The circulation of Pergamon journals grew by 5–10 percent each year during the 1960s, using a strategy of publishing a large number of journals, with the longer-standing journals supporting those that were newly launched until they too became essential. The North American market proved particularly rewarding because of the exchange rate between the U.S. dollar and the British pound. Again, turning to Brian Cox,

> In 1951, when Pergamon was founded, the U.S. dollar had already replaced sterling in the world currency, and until the 1980s remained the benchmark against which all other currencies were measured. Costs and subscription rates grew as journals grew in size and frequency, but were incurred in pounds during many years when the pound fell in value against the dollar—a fact not immediately apparent to librarians in the United States who were pleased with Pergamon's apparently stable prices. The exchange illusion was a major factor in Pergamon's profitability.[10]

The overexpansion of Pergamon resulted in its forced sale in 1991 to Elsevier and the collapse of the Maxwell enterprise. Even the most vehement anticommercial advocate must acknowledge the contribution to publishing made by Pergamon. However, its methods were forcing libraries to address the crisis in journal costs and take action to preserve their ability to offer access to information. Robert Maxwell and other businessmen working from similar premises began to use the notion of "core" journal titles in the literature of science and medicine and the hierarchy of scientific journals that these new bibliographic tools, especially *Science Citation Index*, created to develop new business models. Prices of journals soared. By 1988 the situation had grown serious, and librarian concerns were escalating. Marcia Tuttle's celebrated newsletter *ALA/RTSD Newsletter on Serial Pricing Issues* appeared as a forum in which librarians could document prices and policies as they discovered them, sharing information on details of strategies and marketing within the community.

Competitive commercial publishing increasingly used the strategy of mergers to consolidate markets and increase revenue. With fewer publishers competing in the same business, there would be a larger market share for those who remained. By 2004, the firm of Reed Elsevier owned Lexis Nexis, Martindale Hubbell, Butterworth Harcourt, Holt, Rinehart and Winston,

JAI Press, Chilton, CIS, Academic Press, BioMed Net, Engineering Information, Pergamon Press, Beilstein, Cell Press, Mosby, Churchill, Livingstone Saunders, and of course, Elsevier Science. In 2003, Wolters Kluwer owned CCH, Aspen Publishing, Lippincott Williams and Wilkins, Waverly, Silver Platter, and Ovid. Wolters Kluwer then sold Kluwer Academic Publishers to Candover and Civen, which then merged Kluwer Academic Publishers with Springer Verlag.[11] The benefits publishers received through economies of scale, efficiency, and market share, however, were not reflected in journal prices. Librarians in the United States raised the issue of these large holding companies with the U.S. Department of Justice, but these efforts had no significant impact upon the mergers. Librarians then developed an alternative strategy through the formation of an Information Access Alliance (IAA) of a number of professional associations in the United States, including the Association of Research Libraries, the American Library Association, the Association of College and Research Libraries, the American Association of Law Libraries, the Medical Library Association, and the Scholarly Publishing and Academic Resources Coalition (SPARC). Their cause was a simple one: to demonstrate the direct relationship between the size of the publishing company and price increases and the negative impact of these price increases upon the provision of the results of research to the scholarly and research communities and to the public at large.

The continuing realignments in the world of commercial research publishing and the response on the part of many librarians, the academic community, and the general public was in fact to provoke an international response. The United Kingdom Competition Commission and the European Commission reviewed the business practices of Elsevier and Candover and Civen respectively. In both instances the mergers proceeded. But investigations in the United Kingdom concluded that there was sufficient concern to conduct further investigation into the business practices of science, technical, and medical commercial publishing and marketing.[12] Although the continuing legal debate is unresolved, experimentation in alternative methods of scholarly communication flourishes, in particular the development of noncommercially based scientific publishing alternatives, such as open access.

THE INFLUENCE OF CORE BIBLIOGRAPHIES

Developing a bibliography that is successful creates a tool that allows better access to information; it also affects the nature of the items covered by the bibliography. In effect, it provides those items that are selected for inclusion with visibility and prestige. Garfield's *SCI* brought enhanced visibility and prestige not only to cited authors but also to the journals that were incorporated in the index. One of the early consequences of Garfield's success, therefore, was the transformation of scientific publishing. Instead of a continuous gradient of titles ranging from mediocrity to excellence, there emerged a two-tier structure composed of a minority of titles inside *SCI* corresponding to "core science" and a majority of titles outside (peripheral, marginal, or unnamed science). The pecking order of science had now begun to incorporate a new category—core science—which could easily translate into "elite science."

Decisions to include a title or not into *SCI* seem to have generally been taken in good faith, but this is not the main point: a private company accountable only to itself and its investors had managed to gain a position from where it could affect the visibility, prestige, and authority of any scientific journal. When it is realized how crucial these elements are for any scientific journal, how very central they are for the branding capacity of such journals, it is not difficult to understand the powerful strategic position that the *SCI* now occupied. In itself, this new situation would not have mattered all that much had it limited itself to this result. Some observers, however, were quick to perceive new business possibilities tied to *SCI*'s presence in the world of science. Thanks to Bradford's law, librarians had independently begun to implement selection processes that created collections that were very similar from one institution to another, buying ever more similar materials. It is not surprising, therefore, to see *SCI*'s list of core journals becoming a kind of "must buy" list. Librarians accepted the titles selected by Garfield as a quality filter. As a first approximation, librarians agreed with Garfield's law of concentration of excellence and strove to buy his list. As librarians began increasingly to buy "in step," they contributed to transforming the "must buy" category of titles into an inelastic market, a market where the demand is relatively insensitive to price increases.

Large medical libraries with a mandate to provide access to biomedical research materials certainly were influenced in their collection development by these trends in convergence buying. In addition to the *Science Citation Index*, the *Index Medicus* and its successor, MEDLINE, had an even more powerful effect on identifying core and essential material for medical collections. Any bibliography, unless it is totally comprehensive, will, by its selective nature, define two classes of material—those titles indexed and those titles not indexed. MEDLINE carefully restricts its selection to those titles considered to be the most valuable by an objective and nonpartisan review board of fifteen librarians, scientists, and health professionals known as the Literature Selection Technical Review Committee. It is perhaps redundant to mention that this process is dramatically different from that used to create the *SCI*. The most important criterion for deciding whether to include a title in MEDLINE is the scientific quality of the journal. Journal price and a journal's impact factor are not part of the selection criteria. In 2004, 575,000 articles were indexed from 4,800 journals. Since 1997, MEDLINE has been available over the Internet via PubMed, which also includes other citations that are not part of MEDLINE.[13]

As a publicly funded resource, the MEDLINE database is available free of charge worldwide, with approximately 50 percent of its use being by Americans. Unlike *SCI*, it does not depend on subscriptions and it is not required to show profit. These points may seem obvious yet are worth bearing in mind, since there is one important similarity between these two resources. When a journal is indexed in MEDLINE, it brings to that journal some very significant benefits in addition to prestige: librarians are likely to use indexing in MEDLINE as a criterion for selection, and subscriptions to that title are likely to increase. Once a title is indexed in MEDLINE, both the number and quality of manuscript submissions are likely to increase, as is the amount of advertising revenue. One thing that both MEDLINE and *SCI* have in common is the unintentional consequences of these major services to the medical and scientific community that creates an awesome power to enhance, even to guarantee the success of, a journal.

THE EMERGENCE OF THE ELECTRONIC JOURNAL

The position of the librarian with regard to these developments was extremely difficult. In effect, librarians were caught in a squeeze: if they succeeded in fulfilling their basic mandate to provide good and cost-effective access to the needed medical and scientific literature to their constituency, their libraries became increasingly homogeneous; in fact, they were all buying the same thing. If they lost in the distribution of funds during the budget cycle or if their governing institution had fewer dollars to allocate, they lost the support of their users. If their cries for help went unheeded and they had to resort to cuts in acquisitions and in subscriptions to journals, often the reaction of the academics was to blame librarians for not being capable of doing their job correctly. Rather than look at the general, changing picture of scientific publishing and the pricing patterns of commercial publishers, they might even turn against their immediate colleagues in the administration, especially if they felt the university was not supporting the library infrastructure at a sufficient level to support scientific research.

It is to the credit of members of the library profession that they ultimately managed to address the immediate economic issues around journal cost increases with a variety of institutional and group tactics. But the systemic causes remained poorly identified. It was not in the best interest of the publishers to create transparency regarding their business practices, as we have already seen, and the waters remained muddy. A great deal of "Fear, Uncertainty and Doubt" (FUD)[14] surrounded the question of journal pricing. This had begun in the print era with the debates between librarians and publishers over fixed pricing and became more intense in the electronic era with the bundling of print and electronic subscriptions in the early days of e-journals. It continues into the present with problems of variable pricing between different members of a consortium and among different consortia. No one can deny that these increases in price and profits had been brilliantly engineered and that they rested on a deep understanding of the librarians' quandary: one of their fundamental functions was procuring a basic number of titles at almost any cost in order to provide access to clients' needs. The FUD generated by publishers generally managed to keep anger and revolt at a simmering, and therefore controllable, level. At the same time, and probably because librarians did not succeed in finding lasting solutions to this problem—partially because they also had difficulties in moving beyond symptoms to reach the level of causes—the issue of pricing mesmerized universities for decades, preventing the emergence of suitable strategic alternatives to address the real issues. Much energy was spent, perhaps even wasted, on the pricing issue because it was examined in isolation without much regard to the context and the processes that had brought about this unsustainable publishing system.

The pricing crisis emerged within the print world before anyone seriously contemplated an entirely digital world. Prices began to rise in earnest in the 1970s, although the phenomenon was partially masked by the high rates of inflation that followed the 1973 oil crisis. It became an unavoidable topic in the 1980s, all the more so in that the difficult economic situation of the period put a lot of pressure on university budgets. Academics began to feel the pinch: in poor countries, the transition was drastic, as subscriptions to scientific journals plummeted. In the middle ground of relatively modest institutions in rich or relatively rich countries, cuts in subscriptions affected a sufficiently high percentage of titles to be directly felt by faculty. Librarians bore the brunt of their protests. Only in the richest institutions did the resources more or less rise to the challenge, sufficiently, in any case, to make it a secondary phenomenon for most faculty members. Few librarians were praised for their judicious management during this period.

While prices continued to climb vertiginously, a new phenomenon began to appear at the end of the 1980s and particularly in the early part of the 1990s. The development of the information and communications technologies that we have followed in its broad outline above began to provide new functionalities, new work habits, and a new ethos. It also provided the tools to explore the possibility of shifting the weight of science publishing onto computers and networks. Experiments carried out by a number of individual scientists and academics began to multiply around 1990, some a little before, some a little after. In parallel with the growing number of electronic forums, various experimental forms of electronic journals began to be tested in a number of fields. In the spirit of the Internet, and with the support of the kind of soft money that can be found on occasions to start experiments, these fragile publications were often, in fact most of the time, completely free. They were also much dispersed and, therefore, quite difficult to identify and retrieve. Old hands in this domain may still remember the gallant attempts by a graduate student at the University of Ottawa, Michael Strangelove, to create a list of these forums and experimental publications.[15] Soon, his effort was replaced by the *Directory of Electronic Journals, Newsletters and Academic Discussion Lists*,[16] published by the Association of Research Libraries under the direction of several people, including Ann Okerson, referred to earlier for her significant role in the development of licensing skills among librarians. In the same manner that we should not let ourselves be diverted by pricing issues, we should not remain too long fixated on early experiments in electronic publishing. Important for our purpose here, which is to review the emergence of the open-access movement, is the reaction of publishers, particularly commercial publishers. Publishers moved rapidly to take advantage of the benefits derived from the electronic versions of journals, but a relatively small number of academics were also experimenting with these new tools. In fact, it may well have been this flurry of experiments that alerted the commercial publishers to the fact that they could not treat these digital developments with benign neglect.

Remarkably early, Reed-Elsevier began exploring in earnest how to extend its core business into the digital context. Elsevier's "Tulip"[17] experiment began with a group of large American university libraries in partnership. One of these partners, Princeton, eventually bowed out, but all the other universities stayed on. The basic idea appears now quite naive: Elsevier intended to provide the equivalent of very large CD-ROMs to libraries with both page images and a hidden full text. The hidden full text was there to allow full-text searches. The page images were designed to give the look, if not the feel, of the original print and thereby legitimate these early electronic versions. This method gave rise to files so large that only the bandwidth of an Ethernet campus network could accommodate them comfortably in the early 1990s. Elsevier created digitized texts that resulted in files that were less convenient than the traditional paper version. Printing the page images made the recovery of an article in paper form, which is what most users wanted, an inefficient process.

Ultimately, Elsevier abandoned this technical paraphernalia. Institutional broadband was well developed by the mid-1990s and companies had been remarkably successful in taking advantage of contract law as well as using technical means to monitor and control the use of their product. These developments promoted new approaches to the packaging of electronic journals. Gone were the big CD-ROMs; in their stead came central servers. Libraries only had to subscribe to the titles they wanted on these servers (for a fee) and, as long as they paid, they maintained access. Everything was regulated by the provisions of specific contracts to be negotiated rather than the blanket protection of the copyright terms. Thus, traditional rights such as fair use, or first-sale provision, were no longer automatically acquired by virtue of signing on to a subscription. All had to be negotiated, inch by inch, by librarians, without the benefit of much experience in the finer points of contract law. On the other side, of course, publishers were using experts well versed in contract law. It is one of Ann Okerson's most enduring contributions to the library profession to have succeeded in alerting the library community to the dangers inherent in the new digital context and its licensing schemes. She also began to provide solutions for this new digital context; by analyzing and comparing licenses she emphasized the importance of mastering this new legal environment and its unfamiliar territory. She also underscored the growing need to regroup and create united fronts to face the powerful international publishers.[18]

The debates that began to surround licensing, and then licensing through consortia, have relatively little to do with open access. Nonetheless, the bundling strategies that began to multiply in the 1990s, generally known as "Big Deals," seem to have put a new question to the librarians: what can we do to avoid seeing this new development add itself to the earlier price increases already at work in the print world? This is what was behind the orderly retreat from the Big Deal described in chapter 9. The question was all the more urgent since publishers were using the transition to say two things at once: with digitized materials, we will provide better, richer services; however, these services and their development are very costly and libraries must understand that the transition to the digital era requires a fair amount of financing. Prices continued to escalate, and a number of scholars and scientists began to argue that the solution was indeed an electronic solution. The argument rested on the simple idea that electronic publishing allowed the elimination of printing and mailing and that the server costs were negligible. As many scholarly journals benefit from the support of public money, it even became conceivable that, with electronic publishing, enough money was already in the system to eliminate the subscription model of financing journals altogether and thus make these journals freely accessible.

It is taking some time to separate the issues of electronic publishing and open access, and this distinction is not yet uniformly accepted. For example, offering access within a consortium or on a university campus is easy to mistake for open access, as the results are identical from the users' perspective except in the accounting department. Even librarians have been heard to claim that material ubiquitously available to a group of licensed users under strict licensing terms is "open access." Ironically, the confusion has not been futile, since it has helped to keep alive the issues and visions relating directly to open access. These were to gain full autonomy and momentum in discussions about institutional repositories and optimizing access to scientific information.

THE EMERGENCE OF OPEN ACCESS AND THE RESPONSE OF THE SCIENTIFIC COMMUNITY

The vision of Paul Ginsparg, expressed through the openly available article depository of physics preprints at the Los Alamos National Laboratory, which he started in the summer of 1991,[19] pointed the way to open access at an early stage. Ginsparg's general source of inspiration was the time-honored tradition among physicists of exchanging preprints. He may also have had in mind the older, paper-based Spires system at Stanford University, and he proceeded to transpose it to the Internet. This archive was successful almost from the start, and continues to play an important role in open access. It has inspired a number of similarly organized depositories in various fields, for example Repec in economics.[20] It also forced a number of thorny questions into the open, for example, the issue of association journals coexisting with open-access depositories. In short, its existence has long energized those interested in promoting an open-access agenda. It keeps alive an approach to open access that is based upon depositories of electronic information organized around disciplines. The PubMed Central depository of the National Institutes of Health, which emerged at the end of the decade, is probably the most outstanding example of this disciplinary approach, although its creators emphasize the "public" rather that the "open" aspect of this archive of biomedical information. Its development is discussed in greater detail in chapter 11.

With the possibility of the multiplication of depositories, it became essential to address the question of balkanization and ensuring access in this emerging communications system by developing reliable standards for the exchange of data. Unified search engines seemed a way to enhance the use of these collections of documents, and this, in turn, raised issues of standards, interoperability, and metadata. To begin to address some of these issues, a meeting took place in October 1999 in Santa Fe, New Mexico.[21] This time, the prime movers were the librarians, but computer scientists were involved too. Out of this and subsequent discussions, a new protocol began to emerge, the Open Archives Initiative/Protocol for Metadata Harvesting (OAI/PMH),[22] which in turn gave rise to a series of search engines such as OAISTER.[23]

The development of public or open depositories and the necessary standards for interoperability provided new ways of accessing the literature of science and medicine. The scientific community, most especially the "young Turks," was well aware of these alternatives. Commercial scientific and medical publishers became increasingly concerned with the marketing and profitability of their publications, at times to the detriment of scientific communication. At times, scientific association publishers shared this financial priority as they were often caught in the web of cross subsidization of association activities from the sale of the association's journal. Repeated, sharp debates, facilitated by the presence of numerous Internet forums—an element that certainly played a crucial role in bringing a number of important facts and attitudes to light—increasingly demonstrated the important disconnect between what the researchers and even the public needed and what the publishers were willing to provide. Anger rose, especially when it became obvious that, besides the overt debates, pressure tactics and the threat of legal action were being used to squelch criticism of the dominant commercial model.

The magnitude of this anger can be gauged to some extent by a petition that was launched under the guise of an open letter published by a loose coalition of scientists called the "Public Library of Science" (PloS). Librarians were not part of this "public library"; neither were they invited to join at that particular stage, which focused on scientists only. The document that supported this new approach to a publicly available library of science incorporated many of the points and elements that were to recur with variable intensity over the next few years:

> We support the establishment of an online public library that would provide the full contents of the published record of research and scholarly discourse in medicine and the life sciences in a freely accessible, fully searchable, interlinked form. Establishment of this public library would vastly increase the accessibility and utility of the scientific literature, enhance scientific productivity, and catalyze integration of the disparate communities of knowledge and ideas in biomedical sciences.
>
> We recognize that the publishers of our scientific journals have a legitimate right to a fair financial return for their role in scientific communication. We believe, however, that the permanent, archival record of scientific research and ideas should neither be owned nor controlled by publishers, but should belong to the public and should be freely available through an international online public library.
>
> To encourage the publishers of our journals to support this endeavour, we pledge that, beginning in September 2001, we will publish in, edit or review for, and personally subscribe to only those scholarly and scientific journals that have agreed to grant unrestricted free distribution rights to any and all original research reports that they have published, through PubMed Central and similar online public resources, within 6 months of their initial publication date.[24]

The arguments raised to justify the demands are important: increased accessibility and utility of research results, better scientific productivity, and easier interdisciplinary work—two points that the members of the Weinberg committee in the late 1950s, described earlier (see chapter 6), would have totally agreed with, even though their motives were quite different from those of the PLoS leaders. The concessions are also important to note: the "legitimate right to a fair financial return" is acknowledged and the demands will try to accommodate the business role of the publishers: the six-month delay in freeing the content. Finally, an interesting principle emerges also from this letter: the scientific record belongs to the public. The authors of this letter could have added that it ought to be so because much of this research is financed by public money. Then came the threat: the signatories would no longer cooperate with those who refused these minimal conditions.

Viewed historically, this open letter was a huge failure: the deadline of September 1, 2001, came and went. Publishers sat tight, although a few may have heaved a sigh of relief. As for the signatories, they quickly realized that they did not hold the big end of the stick. From another angle, however, it was a huge success: nearly thirty thousand scientists from all over the world signed this letter, signaling that a new, potentially strong, undercurrent of opinion had managed to mobilize a significant fraction of the biomedical researchers of the world. The petition also received a fair amount of publicity, and the issue began to spill over into media that, normally, do not pay much attention to academic publishing practices. The upshot was that between 1999 and 2001, a number of activities began to converge, revealing a wide variety of participants, but little coordination among them. In fact, in many cases, participants in these various efforts to free the literature of science hardly knew of each other, rendering the move toward open access more like an active, disorganized Brownian motion rather than a single powerful stream. The Budapest Open Access Initiative managed to engineer a more cohesive transformation of this effort.

THE BUDAPEST OPEN-ACCESS INITIATIVE

A variety of individuals were invited to a meeting in Budapest between November 30 and December 1, 2001. Some were from as far away as North and South America, others from Europe, mainly from Britain. All had tickets financed by one organization, George Soros's Open Society Institute (OSI), more precisely, the Information Program of OSI. Two names must be mentioned in this context : Professor Istvan Rev, a historian and archivist of OSI at the Central European University, also funded by George Soros, acting as chair of the Information Programs Board; and Darius Cuplinskas, the Toronto-born Lithuanian who had recently become the director of the newly formed Information Program of the Open Society Institute. Also present, besides programs staff were members of another organization also initiated by OSI: eIFl.net—a consortium of libraries from "Transition and Third World" countries, mainly located in the former Soviet Union and in parts of Asia and in Africa.

Ten out of the sixteen attendees were not associated with OSI but were familiar with each other's work, having come across each other through conferences and discussion lists where open access was being discussed and debated. There were some very strong egos in that room, and tempers nearly flared on a number of occasions. Clearly, this was not the usual group of academics or librarians. Although suits and ties were sported by a few attendees, academic reserve was never a favored form of behavior in this particular collective. A number of the invitees were particularly articulate and energetic people: Michael Eisen from the Public Library of Science, Stevan Harnad, and Peter Suber.[25]

What was at stake was simple: OSI's Information Program had taken notice of the swirling of ideas in the area of open access and was exploring the possibility of supporting this intriguing development. Like everybody else, OSI members were trying to make sense of the various calls for action and cries of indignation that attendees knew well. The role of publishers was still a big concern in this particular setting, as was the anxious voice of librarians. Librarians played a formative role in developing a place for open access within the Information Program. The Information Program had been organized out of earlier programs, one of which was a library program, eIFL.net. Among the people assembled in Budapest, several were librarians or very familiar with library issues.

The discussions in the Budapest meeting revealed the existence of two markedly different approaches to open access: on the one hand, many advocated the creation or transformation of existing journals into open-access publications, leaving for later the issue of how to finance this model. Others favored depositories of articles and self-archiving. Stevan Harnad had already fully articulated this side of the issue. The scene was also complicated by the fact that side issues continued to emerge during the discussions. For example, one attendee wanted to reform the peer-review process and make it a paying proposition as a way to build a new and original business plan. Other attendees were raising questions with the Third World in mind. Still other attendees were trying to work out the economics of open-access journals and, to some extent, the economics of archives, be they based on disciplines or institutions. The librarians and the publishers had a strong commitment to journals and journal titles: this is after all the bread and butter of their respective (and symmetrical) business. Rick Johnson, director of the SPARC initiative, was deeply involved in creating competition for the existing, overpriced journals, and the idea of creating open-access journals sounded extremely good. This was, after all, the idea of competition pushed to its extreme; to him and several others, it brought to mind the way free software had challenged the de facto monopoly established by Microsoft. Reining in the big publishers seemed feasible through open access—a point of view shared by Jan Velterop, another invitee, who, at the time, worked for the open-access commercial publisher, Biomed Central.[26]

Scientists and scholars, on the other hand, were more ambivalent on the problem. While access to the literature was obviously of the essence to them, the branding capacity of journals was equally important. For this reason, that particular group was more divided. No one knew at the time that the Public Library of Science was going to emerge anew from its spectacular failure—a failure, as we have seen, that was so visible. It was to achieve spectacular success in a series of open-access publications fueled by an important grant of nine million dollars (U.S.) from the Gordon and Betty Moore Foundation. With this large lump sum, the new PLoS began to create a series of journals modeled after the business recipe tested first by Biomed Central—the author(s) or (more probably) a substitute pays up front for the cost of handling the manuscript prior to publication. PLoS also pushed extremely hard for the highest possible impact factor so as to demonstrate that an open-access journal can have impact factors equal or superior to the best toll-gated publications.[27] PLoS is discussed in more detail in chapter 11.

In parallel, other scientists, particularly Stevan Harnad, argued that open access had nothing to do with publishers; all that was needed was the decision by scientists to self-archive some version of their own papers in such a way as to make it equivalent to the published/refereed version. The important point to recognize here is that the term "archive" is not used in its technical sense but rather to mean the availability of an author's work in open and digital form in a manner that permits it to be harvested with the use of the recent Open Archives Initiative/Protocol for Metadata Harvesting. For Stevan Harnad, therefore, all that was needed was a limited amount of financial support on the part of the research institutions, universities, and research laboratories and open access could be achieved. In this particular scenario of self-archiving, open access could be achieved without worrying about existing journals and their complex economic underpinnings.

The discussion circled around these issues, and, for the most part, most of the protagonists stayed on their respective positions. At the end of the day, however, the group found itself faced by a looming deadline of airplane schedules and the need to return home. No resolution as to the proper way to achieve open access most efficiently seemed to be nearer. At that point, it was suggested that if nothing more came out of this meeting, at least some sort of coherent statement should reflect the commonalities of concerns and project to the world the importance of open access for future development. Thus was born the idea of a kind of manifesto that would carry the message forward. In the minds of a few, the very idea of drafting a manifesto was also viewed as a way to maintain the momentum of the group and to force it as much as possible to come to some sort of closure about defining a clear objective and clear means to achieve it.

It took more than ten weeks to achieve this and the process that led to the final result was in good part due to the extraordinary analytical and writing ability of one of the attendees, the philosopher Peter Suber. He did not write the Budapest Open Access Initiative; just about all the attendees introduced additions, emendations, and interesting formulations on various facets of the declaration, but the general framework, the tone, and the clarity of the exposition would not have been what they came to be, had not Peter Suber brought to bear his talent for the right word and the clear argument that one still finds every day in his blog on open access. BOAI, as it has come to be known, begins with language that is both prophetic and literary:

> An old tradition and a new technology have converged to make possible an unprecedented public good. The old tradition is the willingness of scientists and scholars to publish the fruits of their research in scholarly journals without payment, for the sake of inquiry and knowledge. The new technology is the internet. The public good they make possible is the world-wide electronic distribution of the peer-reviewed journal literature and completely free and unrestricted access to it by all scientists, scholars, teachers, students, and other curious minds. Removing access barriers to this literature will accelerate research, enrich education, share the learning of the rich with the poor and the poor with the rich, make this literature as useful as it can be, and lay the foundation for uniting humanity.[28]

The last point was a vision: making possible a movement toward knowledge that would help humanity become ever more conscious of all that supports its unity. This was not quite the "world brain" of H. G. Wells, although it too found its roots in libraries, encyclopedias, and their potential,[29] and certainly not the mysterious flow of ideas from brain to brain of the idealists; rather it sees humanity carrying some sort of common purpose in the tension that exists, through conversation, between collaboration and competition. The use of the word "initiative" in the phrase "Budapest Open Access Initiative" was derived from the realistic expectation that this "initiative" would be accompanied by solid funding to allow the exploration and testing of this initiative. The OSI Information Program was committing itself to spending about three million dollars over three years to promote open access. The loftiness of the goals and the financial commitment converged to create a strong message that was heard in many quarters, especially as it was echoed by the press in many parts of the world.[30]

The publication and wide distribution of BOAI quickly led to a flurry of activities, too numerous to recount here.[31] Taken together, they show a growing consciousness for strategic considerations that enhance the deployment of open-access archives and of open-access journals. For example, the Joint Information Systems Committee (JISC), a British institution promoting the use of new technologies to enhance higher education, began to finance a number of projects that were supporting the progression toward open access in ancillary ways. JISC initiated the Romeo (Rights MEtadata for Open Achiving) project. This project was looking at intellectual property issues surrounding and potentially threatening the practice of self-archiving that was advocated in BOAI. Romeo produced an analysis of publishers after studying carefully their rights transfer contracts with authors. This important work may have ultimately contributed to persuading many publishers to accept some form of self-archiving by authors. These publishers are nowadays characterized as displaying various shades of green.[32] JISC also investigated issues of preservation and the building of depositories.[33] In Holland, the Dutch equivalent to JISC, SURF,[34] began to act in a parallel way. Two years later, JISC and SURF would begin hosting joint meetings to benefit from each others' experience and knowledge. Similar developments began being discussed, planned, and ultimately implemented to some extent in a variety of countries in the industrialized world. However, this was not going to be the end of the BOAI's impact.

More important was that BOAI managed to attract the attention of a number of important institutions that finance research in various countries in the world. Most prominent among those were the Howard Hughes Foundation and NIH in the United States, the Wellcome Trust in Britain, the Max Planck Gesellschaft in Germany, and INSERM and CNRS in France, to name the better-known ones.

THE MEDICAL LIBRARY
ASSOCIATION REACTS TO OPEN ACCESS

The leadership of the Medical Library Association has expressed its position on open access in the pages of the *Journal of the Medical Library Association*. In 2004, the position of the association was clearly expressed by T. Scott Plutchak,[35] editor of the *Journal of the Medical Library Association* and Patricia Thibodeau, chair of the association's Task Force on Scholarly Publishing and MLA immediate past president. Plutchak describes how the relationship between librarians and publishers has deteriorated over the past decades. The deterioration of understanding between publishers and medical librarians had been discussed in relation to the correspondence generated by Peter Stangl in the pre-Internet era. Plutchak sees the early years of this century as a period of increasing acrimony, the result of ever increasing subscription costs far greater than inflationary increases compounded with the complexities of various Big Deal licensing schemes. These schemes have increased the workload of librarians, Plutchak argues, and have served to fuel the belief that publishers are "rapacious, predatory entities, determined to squeeze the last dollar from libraries, no matter what the cost to society." But he also makes the important point that not all publishers are the same, nor should they be treated in the same manner, noting the enthusiastic support of medical librarians for *PLoS Biology*. (*PLoS Medicine* had not yet been published at the time of this editorial.) The essence of his editorial is concerned with the question of what constitutes a fair price, and he raises the issue of whether an institution should pay more for a subscription simply because its readership increases in the electronic age. Recall the definition of public goods in chapter 1 in which these products are defined as any commodity that can be extended to a greater number of people at no additional cost.

A second concern is the practice of cross-subsidization by association publishers when revenue generated by the sale of journal subscriptions is used to support other member services such as the cost of annual meetings. This is not an issue in commercial publishing, where the purpose is to maximize net revenue from sales. Given these problems, Plutchak finds it perfectly natural that medical librarians would rush forth to embrace the open-access movement. However, his basic argument for open access is more powerful than these concerns. In making it, he articulates a fundamental value of medical librarians when he writes that the reason to support the open-access movement is that "it promises to be a very good thing for society." Here he acknowledges the responsibility of the librarian to provide access to information for all who need it and support those strategies and changes in a larger society that make this possible. Interestingly, he is not particularly enthusiastic about the general potential of open access to unlock the medical literature on behalf of the public at large. What ignites his support is improved access to clinical medical information by the health care practitioner in rural America. Nor is Plutchak happy with compromises that make the medical literature available six months or a year after it is first published. His reasons for embracing open access are deeply grounded in a sense of social responsibility, and as a citizen he has no hesitation in supporting the movement. As a practicing medical librarian, he is well aware of the price that must be paid, metaphorically speaking, in the transition to open access. All things considered, he speculates on whether in the final analysis, it really will be cheaper. But he has no doubt that it will be better! Supporting open access may promise to relieve the pressure on library budgets, but this alone does not provide the reason. Librarians must consider the impact on the way libraries are managed and the role of librarians in lending their strength to the open-access initiative. A return to fundamental values will be part of the landscape when access to medical information is no longer determined by the size of the library budget.

In 2004, Patricia Thibodeau, a past president of the Medical Library Association, addressed the question of open access.[36] The approach to the issue was somewhat unusual. The question of open access had arisen at a business meeting of the association during the annual spring meeting through a proposal to reject support of the association from publishers who did not support open access. This was a complicated issue because it addressed not only the relationship between publishers and their subscribers but also the financing of the association. The membership asked the executive of the association to study the issue and determine appropriate action at its next board meeting in September. In analyzing the situation, it became clear that if implemented, the resolution would jeopardize finances, since MLA received approximately 37 percent of its finances from all publishers. Further, it was seen to be difficult to determine what publishers actually supported open access. There was also the added threat, in a profession not known to be overpaid, that the membership fees and registration at the annual meeting would need to increase to compensate for the loss of publisher income. The result was that the board of the association did not support the resolution because there was seen to be a "current lack of clarity about what constitutes open access."[37] This was an interesting result, as it demonstrates the challenge professional organizations, including library organizations, face in their funding models. Cross subsidization through revenue received from the rental of exhibition space to publishers is, in this instance, in a category similar to the revenue received from subscriptions to journals published by associations. When publishers of journals using traditional subscription-based models of publication and sales consider open access, the inevitable question becomes one of an alternative source of revenue to replace that which is lost to the association as a whole. This is an understandable response and one that any financially responsible association executive must make. However, the result is confusion in the true costs of the journal. The Medical Library Association has created an open-access portal to monitor the situation as a result of these discussions. Included are letters of advocacy in support of legislation.[38]

Plutchak undertook a detailed study of the impact of open access of the *Journal of the Medical Library Association* on membership in the Medical Library Association. Like many professional societies, the Medical Library Association provides copies of its journal to paying members of the association. In June 2001, recent years of the *Journal of the Medical Library Association* became openly accessible within PubMed Central, and by November 2003, the entire back file to 1911 was available. Plutchak concludes that this initiative did not have a significant impact on the membership of the association and that the greatly increased readership of the *Journal* reported by PMC was seen as a definite benefit to the association.[39] The Medical Library Association is typical of many medium-sized professional associations. With an annual budget of three million dollars, approximately 5 percent is allocated to the production of the *Journal*, which generates revenue of some forty thousand dollars after expenses. Like other associations, the MLA cross-subsidizes other activities of the association with revenue generated by the *Journal*. A survey of the members of the association indicated that 61 percent of the members felt that free availability made no difference in their decision to become a member; only 5 percent felt that they would be less likely to become members because the *Journal* was freely available on the Internet. One particularly interesting finding was that 30 percent of the members surveyed felt that they would be more likely to renew their membership due to the Internet availability of the *Journal*.

LIBRARIES AND OPEN ACCESS: INSTITUTIONAL RESPONSIBILITY AND INSTITUTIONAL REPOSITORIES

Open access rests on a belief that information is a public good and that in the information age, a digital bird need know no cage. Thus far in this review of the origins and development of open access, librarians have been part of our story largely as a result of their reactions to the high costs of providing access to scientific and medical journals. As we have seen, they were not part of the PLoS initiative. Open access is a process of research and publication, and as such, involves primarily the researcher and the publisher. The discussions, indeed the heated debates, that have taken place regarding the ways in which open availability of the literature can be accomplished have been led by the researchers themselves. The ways of promoting open access that have been identified have included the development of journals published in open access and made freely available over the Internet and the use of self-archiving by the researcher to make the publications of an individual researcher available through the initiative of the individual researcher. The engagement of the librarian is not fundamental to either of these alternatives. Yet the librarian community has been intensely engaged in discussions of these alternatives, and is playing an essential role in the development of institutional repositories.

The development of institutional repositories is often linked to the idea of open access. Indeed, at some professional librarian meetings the acronyms "OA" and "IR" are seldom heard independent of each other. This suggests the important emerging role that the librarian is able to play in developing access to information in the public space. But it is possible for an institution to maintain a repository that provides access to its contents to members of the institution and to other selected groups, without making the contents publicly available. As institutions came to do more and more of their business—writing, teaching, publishing, communicating, and governing—in digital form, institutions assumed new responsibilities for managing the change from analog to digital, including the need to preserve the digital record and to migrate content to ensure the preservation of the digital record. The need for an available and secure record of the business of the university, in the fullest sense of the term, became apparent to leaders at most research and teaching institutes. The institutional repository represented "a recognition that the intellectual life and scholarship of our universities will increasingly be represented, documented, and shared in digital form, and that a primary responsibility of our universities is to exercise stewardship over these riches: both to make them available and to preserve them."[40] There is nothing in this definition that requires that the information in an institution's repository be made publicly available to all who wish to access it. Yet as librarians begin to address the need to work collaboratively within their institutions to establish the institutional repositories, it is with the understanding that these repositories will be open. Institutional repositories, as their name indicates, are the result of the acceptance of the need and the responsibility of the institution to provide secure and accessible access to digital content created at the institution. Policies that govern the repository will therefore be the result of institutional practice and needs. Institutional repositories serve a need quite different from that of disciplinary repositories serving, for example, physics, perhaps the best known example.

Librarians are increasingly involved in the creation of repositories as it becomes clear that the development of institutional repositories is essential to access and preservation of research and scholarship in the digital age. Some researchers see the repository as a means of extending their visibility and enhancing the use of their publications through deposit in a secure and openly accessible server. Others, more familiar with the economics of scholarly publishing, may see digital publishing and the deposit of their work in repositories as a means of repatriating publishing from the commercial environment to the academy. For their part, librarians are experimenting with digital repositories as a means of serving institutional and academic needs simultaneously. Eight large university libraries in the United States, Canada, and England launched the DSpace Federation in 2003 with a grant from the Andrew W. Mellon Foundation.[41] At each institution a repository was developed using the software developed by MIT, called DSpace, and an institutional initiative encouraged faculty to deposit their research data, publications, and learning objects in the institutions' digital repository. Space in the institutional repository is made available for the deposit of digital materials and for searching all or part of the material deposited by the various communities of the member university. The content is indexed by Google, which searches institutional servers where the content resides. It is highly visible in Google as well as reliable. As a result, the visibility of the researcher is increased.

Despite these evident advantages, these repositories are not growing rapidly. Participation is voluntary, and many researchers need to be encouraged to include their work. At least one administrator of a repository has contemplated the payment of faculty to deposit their publications! Support is offered by the library staff to convert material for deposit, to add metadata to describe the document, and to clear copyright. The benefit of long-term preservation of the digital document and enhanced access is clearly understood. More than one writer has speculated on why institutional repositories have been developing so slowly.[42] The fundamental reason is that scientific communication is deeply grounded in the discipline. The identity of the researcher is based in his discipline and only secondarily in his institution. Any activity that does not promote or relate to the discipline is likely to be a low priority to the productive researcher. If the individual scientist sees the repository as a means of extending access to research in the discipline and of enhancing visibility in the discipline, participation is far more likely. The phenomenal success of the physics archive of Paul Ginsparg illustrates this point. The importance of subject archives is the key to the success of the repository. The institutional repository may serve a dual purpose—to the researcher and his particular discipline and to the institution, but the repository must be seen as part of the advancement of the discipline and scholarly communication. In the next chapter the success of one particular disciplinary archive in the public domain, PubMed Central, will be explored along with the factors that presently limit the realization of its full success.

NOTES

1. Derek J. de Solla Price, *Little Science, Big Science* (New York: Columbia University Press, 1963).
2. Robert K. Merton, *The Sociology of Science: Theoretical and Empirical Investigations* (Chicago: University of Chicago Press, 1973).
3. William D. Garvey, *Communication: The Essence of Science* (Oxford: Pergamon Press, 1979).
4. Joseph C. Donohue, *Understanding Scientific Literatures: A Bibliometric Approach* (Cambridge, MA: MIT Press: 1973).
5. Samuel C. Bradford, "Sources of Information on Specific Subjects," *Engineering* 137 (January 26, 1934): 85–86.
6. Paul Wouters, *The Citation Culture* (Amsterdam: Academisch Proefschrift doctor aan de Universiteit van Amsterdam, 1999), 22.
7. Brian Cox, "The Pergamon Phenomenon 1951–1991: Robert Maxwell and Scientific Publishing," *Learned Publishing* 15, no. 4 (2002): 274.
8. Brian Cox explains, "Before [WWII], most STM English-language books and journals had been published by learned societies and were almost exclusively devoted to works for their members. War-impelled research far outstripped the capacity of this genteel publishing. A new breed of publishers saw the commercial possibilities in a business that, they foresaw correctly, would set enviable standards of growth and profitability in the succeeding decades." Cox, "The Pergamon Phenomenon," 273.
9. See http://www.garfield.library.upenn.edu/papers/history/heritagey1998 .html (accessed November 30, 2005).
10. Cox, "The Pergamon Phenomenon," 276.
11. Mary M. Case, "Information Access Alliance: Challenging Competitive Behavior in Academic Publishing," *College and Research Library News* 65, no. 6 (June 2004): 314–16.
12. See http://www.antitrust.institute.org (accessed November 30, 2005).
13. Sheldon Kotzin, "Journal Selection for MEDLINE," World Library and Information Congress; 71st IFLA General Conference and Council, Health and Biosciences Libraries, http://www.ifla.org/IV/ifla71/Programme.htm (accessed August 31, 2005).
14. This form of disinformation has emerged in the context of the debates surrounding free software. Arguments playing on peripheral phenomena, such as cur-

rency exchange rates, were often introduced in the discussions, as has been mentioned earlier.

15. A copy of this early effort remains available on a German site: http://www .heise.de/ix/raven/Literature/Journals/ElJournals.html (accessed September 1, 2005).

16. Association of Research Libraries, *Directory of Electronic Journals, Newsletters, and Academic Discussion Lists* (Washington, DC: Association of Research Libraries).

17. Tulip stands for "The University Licensing Program." The word "licensing" was, therefore, present as early as 1991 in the Elsevier experiment in electronic publishing.

18. Licensing at Elsevier started in 1996. Liblicense-l began the same year.

19. For a brief analysis of this disciplinary depository, with some historical details, see Paul Ginsparg, "Winners and Losers in the Global Research Village," http:// arxiv.org/blurb/pg96unesco.html (accessed September 1, 2005).

20. Repec or "Research Papers in Economics," http://repec.org/ (accessed September 1, 2005).

21. See http://www.ecs.soton.ac.uk/~harnad/Hypermail/Amsci/0421.html (accessed September 1, 2005).

22. Open Archive Initiative—Protocol for Metadata Harvesting. The term "open" is used here in the computer science meaning of interoperable. Much confusion has surrounded this term, as few realized that it could be applied to completely toll-gated collections. See http://www.openarchives.org/ (accessed September 1, 2005).

23. See http://oaister.umdl.umich.edu/o/oaister/ (accessed September 1, 2005).

24. See http://www.plos.org/about/letter.html (accessed September 1, 2005).

25. The list of attendees corresponds to the list of the initial signatories to the Budapest Open Access Initiative.

26. Jan Velterop resigned from Biomed Central in the spring of 2005. He now leads the "open choice" group at the reincarnation of Springer, which took place when Candover and Cinven bought Kluwer and Springer and placed the new merged company under the guidance of Derk Haank, the former CEO at Reed-Elsevier.

27. The very first measure of *PloS Biology*'s impact factor was 13.9. The expectation is that it will grow further because PloS journals are just beginning and it will take some time before their impact factors begin to plateau.

28. See http://www.earlham.edu/~peters/fos/fosblog.html For Peter Suber's description of the December meeting in Budapest, see http://www.earlham.edu/ ~peters/fos/newsletter/12-05-01.htm (accessed November 30, 2005).

29. See http://sherlock.berkeley.edu/wells/world_brain.html for Wells's original text of 1937, first published in the *Encyclopédie française*, and then reprinted in English in a volume of essays called *World Brain* (accessed November 30, 2005).

30. For one example, see http://www.upi.com/view.cfm?StoryID=12022002-031227-9710r (accessed November 30, 2005).

31. Peter Suber's "Timeline of the Open Access Movement" gives a clear image of the numerous pieces of news related to OA after February 14, 2002.

32. See http://www.sherpa.ac.uk/romeo.php (accessed November 30, 2005).

33. See http://tardis.eprints.org/ (accessed November 30, 2005).

34. See http://www.surf.nl/en/oversurf/index.php (accessed November 30, 2005).

35. T. Scott Plutchak, "Embracing Open Access," *Journal of the Medical Library Association* 92, no. 3 (January 2004): 1–3.

36. Patricia Thibodeau, "Advocating for Open Access," *MLA News* no. 371 (November–December 2004): 24.

37. Thibodeau, "Advocating for Open Access," 1.

38. See http://www.mlanet.org/government/info_access/ (accessed November 30, 2005).

39. T. Scott Plutchak, "The Impact of Open Access for the *Journal of the Medical Library Association*." Paper presented at the ninth World Congress on Health Information and Libraries, Salvador de Bahia, Brazil (September 23, 2005): 19.

40. Clifford A. Lynch, "Institutional Repositories: Essential Infrastructure for Scholarship in the Digital Age," *ARL, a Bimonthly Report on Research Library Issues and Actions from ARL, CNI, and Sparc* 226 (February 2003): 3.

41. See www.dspace.org/federation (accessed December 8, 2005).

42. See, as an example, Leslie Chan, "Supporting and Enhancing Scholarship in the Digital Age: The Role of Open-Access Institutional Repositories," *Canadian Journal of Communication* 29 (2004): 277–300.

11

NEW SOLUTIONS IN ACCESS TO MEDICAL INFORMATION

The two preceding chapters provided background on the emergence of open access, with its deep roots in technology and scientific communication, and on the accelerated economic crisis in providing access to the journal literature in the digital era. This chapter is an attempt to answer the question of whether there is a better way of providing access to medical information. The answer to this question is quite simply, "yes." But the question is not simple; it involves a system of scholarly communication that is more than three hundred and fifty years old. We have already seen that the cast of characters involved is staggeringly large: medical and scientific researchers, university administrators, librarians, publishers, and the reading public, to say nothing of a formidable group of scholars worldwide, probably about one hundred in number, who have made the subject of alternative methods in scholarly communication and publishing the focus of their own research interests. Another complexity is the need to refine the question of whether there is a better way by asking the follow-up question, "Better for whom?"

In this chapter we shall take a very brief look at the established system of scholarly communication in science as it has evolved over three and a half centuries. Some apology is due for yet again visiting this subject, with so much written on this topic, especially in the past thirty years as the dominance of scientific journals from the larger commercial publishing houses became evident and prices skyrocketed. However, it is not possible to evaluate alternative methods in scholarly communication without understanding the roots of the system, the different interest groups, and what those groups have at stake in the established system. Finally, we shall examine a number of alternatives to the dominant system of scholarly communication that have been developed in the past decade and attempt to evaluate them as well as we can in a rapidly changing environment. The word "sustainable" will be used both to defend and to criticize the dominant method of publication: we shall see how some members of the cast of thousands claim that these new alternatives are not sustainable because they allegedly threaten the assurance of the peer-review system and the well-established structure of the journal. On the opposite side of the debate, advocates of alternatives to the commercially based models claim that the present dominant model is not sustainable for economic reasons. Finally, a word about why all this is important to medical librarians. Throughout this book we have seen demonstrated the core value of medical librarians in providing access to medical information to all who need to use it. Over more than a century of specialization, medical librarians have affirmed their commitment to this core value in their professional lives. They have seen their ability to act in the interests of users curtailed by the present dominant medical publishing methods and have taken a stand on this issue. In doing so, they have become part of the cast of characters that will play out this drama to its uncertain conclusion. As we shall see, a large number of the alternatives to the present system have been incubated within the medical community and the agencies that fund medical research.

Since the work of the Medical Library Association in the 1930s, described earlier in this work, medical librarians have been engaged in the question of the cost of medical and scientific journals and its impact on providing access to the medical literature. In the Internet era, governments, scientific organizations, and universities have developed the robust networks necessary to the access of electronic information. And medical and scientific publishers have transformed their communication and production systems in the digital era to produce the e-journal. Despite these major advances, many medical librarians are engaged in a process to reshape the system of distribution of the published results of medical and scientific investigation as it is presently determined by major commercial publishers. They are not alone. Why is this effort gaining momentum? The unprecedented advances in providing information access in the Internet era have also created the possibility of improved ways of providing access to the medical and research communities worldwide. In the chapter on consumer and patient information, we have seen the unparalleled progress patients and their families have made in learning about their illness, made possible by advances in information technology. And we have also seen the growth of access to clinical information when and where it is of most benefit to the health care professional. But the issues of ownership of this information and its accompanying control through copyright continue to place constraints on information access. The Internet and globalization have created a new world that impacts on virtually (no pun intended) every aspect of life.

The arrival of electronic publishing is frequently compared in significance to the invention of printing in the fifteenth century. In his definitive study of the history of scientific publishing, David Kronick describes the multidimensional factors that contributed to the blossoming of scientific journals after the advent of printing. David Kronick was a skilled medical library administrator whose career in medical libraries predated the arrival of the Internet; nonetheless, like many of the earlier leaders in the profession, he has provided a convincing justification for looking at medical information in the broader context of scientific communication rather than focusing only on publishing.

The changes that helped to create a favorable environment in which the scientific periodical could develop were not entirely intellectual. They were social, economic, and political as well. There was, of course, an articulate and leisured class in the Middle Ages that could have provided a potential audience for the periodical, but it was only with the economic expansion of the fifteenth and sixteenth centuries that this class was considerably increased, and what was more significant, its character changed. One of the important prerequisites for the existence of any medium of communication is an audience.[1] Kronick's expanded view of the environment that helped to stimulate the development of the scientific journal in the seventeenth century includes a growing literate public as part of the readership of the journals. The parallel to today is clear in the literate lay public (consumers of health services) who are creating demands for access to the medical literature.

We have argued that certain economic solutions for providing access to scientific journals, in particular the Big Deal, are not economically or intellectually sustainable in the long term. But these arguments from the academy, originating with researchers, administrators, and librarians, may not be sufficiently compelling for some readers. We need to turn to the needs of patients in the health care system, the public at large, and heath care workers in less-developed countries to hear a growing voice for improved and affordable access to the medical literature. The number of participants in the growing debate over new models of scientific communication in the digital age adds complexity. Another challenge is the long and successful history of scientific and medical publishing in journals, admirably described by Kronick, on which the present system is building. When Henry Oldenburg, secretary to the Royal Society, created *The Philosophical Transactions* of the Royal Society of London in 1665, he was establishing the bedrock on which medical and scientific publishing was to build. The *Phil Trans*, as this publication came to be known, "aimed at creating a public record of original contributions to knowledge . . . helping to validate original knowledge."[2] The *Phil Trans* established precedence and original thinking in medicine and natural philosophy, as the sciences were known at the time of the journal's founding. The publishing of papers not only created a scholarly record, it also helped to formalize a hierarchy based upon primacy of discovery as evidenced in published results. Certainly it was a watershed in the development of the scientific journal.

Who read the *Phil Trans*? Obviously, members of the Royal Society were a primary audience. But scientific communities and specialties were not fixed categories during the period of the scientific revolution. Determining readership is never an easy task. We know from book plates who had access to information through ownership, but who read without owning and who owned without plating? Science had yet to be professionalized and specialized to the extent that those who were not specialists would not be able to comprehend an article on natural history, an experiment on the mechanics of breathing, or the physiology of an insect. Experiments by Robert Hooke and other natural philosophers could be comprehended by the educated layperson and could be replicated in drawing rooms as entertainments by the lay scientist. The number of university-trained physicians and scientists was small, and the scientific journal could reach a general audience.[3]

During the period of the scientific revolution and continuing into the Enlightenment, natural philosophy, including physiology and medicine, enjoyed a great popularity among the literate general public. In our own time the lay reader of medical articles reemerges in the issues surrounding patient and consumer health information. This is especially true with respect to the expert patient, the literate patient, or family member who is well informed not only through the literature for patients but by reading the professional medical literature. It is yet another of history's ironies that during the period when literacy rates were low, in the seventeenth century, the literate public read easily the literature of science and medicine. Today, in the developed world where universal literacy is attainable, the public has difficulty obtaining access to the professional literature of science and medicine. Today's debates over open access are about unlocking the literature that is at present "toll gated" and making it available to all who are able to read it.

The *Phil Trans* defined the beginning of the scientific journal and the stimulation of scientific investigation and communication that was to foster a number of journals, proceedings, reviews, and other collections in medicine and science. Kronick has estimated that the number of these publications increased from 30 in 1699 to 1,052 in 1790.[4] This was a sizable increase but not yet at the level of the exponential growth that has been documented by Price.[5] Exponential growth of the journal literature fueled the development of the great abstracting and indexing services that were needed to control the rapidly growing literature. It also was the reason for the flourishing of the great European scientific publishing houses that provide the basis of international commercial publishing in science, technology, and medicine (STM). Today Elsevier Publishing is a model of this growth in the publishing industry. In 2003, the firm of Reed Elsevier accounted for more than 25 percent of the world market in STM publishing.[6] But although Elsevier is among the oldest and by far the largest corporation dating from 1880, when the present firm of Elsevier was established in Rotterdam by Jacobus George Robbers, there is no continuity between today's company founded by Robbers and the historic Elzevier House of the late sixteenth century. Lodewijk Elzevier had moved his publishing business to Leiden where the university had been established in 1575, and Lodewijk and his descendants found the proximity to the university good for business. The House of Elzevier was very much a university publishing house and continued in business until 1712. When Robbers established his scientific publishing house, he chose to use both the elm tree and hermit logo with the moto "non solus," and the name of the earlier firm, with a slightly modified spelling.[7]

THE EMERGING ALTERNATIVE

Even a relatively superficial understanding of the history of scientific communication provides insight into the reasons that change is both difficult and controversial for all those engaged in it. Adapting information systems and technology to publishing and to libraries was challenging but, by comparison, relatively simple. The purpose and the product were still the same, although the medium changed. On the other hand, a journal in electronic form made possible entirely new ways of communicating. More than a quarter of a century ago, Meadows envisioned the idea of a repository as a way of improving communication in science and recognized the conceptual shift that would be necessary to achieve it as well as the need for government to engage.

> An effective central depository might well require some element of financing by the state—an involvement which many learned societies and

publishers would regard with some suspicion. However, other journal concepts currently under discussion which is more radical . . . do ultimately depend upon government funds. The most striking example is the "electronic journal." The intention of this type of "journal" is that the "papers" should be input directly into computers housed in the authors' institutions. These papers are them made available via the computer network to other people on the journal circulation list. The computer draws the attention of readers to the appearance of each new paper and they can decide for themselves whether they wish to call it up for more detailed study.[8]

Meadows's vision of a "central depository" of research articles anticipates some of the contemporary development in institutional repositories described in the preceding chapter, although it is a far cry from the repository that is emerging today. What both Meadows and today's repository share is an approach to the journal article that is direct rather than one that moves from journal to article.

CHANGING THE SYSTEM: THE SCHOLARLY PUBLISHING AND ACADEMIC RESOURCES COALITION

The idea of alternative publications to counterbalance the dominant commercial titles was present in the Scholarly Publishing and Academic Resources Coalition (SPARC) initiative, although journals published by SPARC, unlike the Public Library of Science titles, are neither free nor freely available. The SPARC initiative arose in 1997 at the Annual Meeting of the Association of Research Libraries. Fatigued by the relentless increases in the cost of scientific journals and the inability to meet user needs as a result, Kenneth Frazier, director of libraries at the University of Wisconsin, made the following grassroots proposal to the membership of the Association:

> The question I keep finding myself returning to is, what are we really going to do to address the issue? I would like to suggest that we need to develop a fund in order to create new publication models. There is no way around it. If 100 institutions would put up $10,000 each to fund 10 start-up journals that would compete back to back with the most expensive scientific and technical journals to which we currently subscribe, we would have $100,000 a year available for each of those 10 start-up titles. . . . This amount of money, by the way, is smaller than the an-

nual increase that we are now experiencing for the most expensive journal list to which we subscribe. Such an endeavor would cost us less than the price of these subscriptions per year.[9]

Each institutional member of the association was asked to provide an initial financial contribution as seed money for the development of an alternative model. Frazier's creative challenge to the membership was rooted in strong principles of providing access to information to all who need to use it. From its inception, SPARC was designed to create new models and to advocate for change in scholarly publishing. Despite its genesis in the frustration over the costs of medical and scientific journals, SPARC was neither reactive nor negative. Founding members saw SPARC as a means to exploit fully the revolutionary potential of the digital age. Its purpose was the development of alternative methods of scholarly communication and a dedication to changing the old system that had become focused on high profit margins.

Established in 2002 under the leadership of Rick Johnson, its founding director, today SPARC is "an international alliance of libraries igniting change in scholarly communication. . . . It pursues this goal through three initiatives:

> *Incubation*: SPARC creates and develops competitive alternatives to current high priced commercial journals and digital aggregations. . . .
>
> *Advocacy*: SPARC promotes fundamental changes in the system of scholarly communication. . . . The advocacy thrust leverages the impact of SPARC's publishing partnerships, providing broad awareness of the possibilities for change and emboldening scholars to act.
>
> *Education*: SPARC develops campaigns aimed at enhancing awareness of scholarly communication issues and supports expanded institutional and community participation in and control over the scholarly communication process.[10]

SPARC is flourishing, fueled by annual membership dues, the commitment of members to purchase scientific publishing initiatives funded by the SPARC initiative, and a series of strategic alliances with public interest groups, certain scientific societies, and affiliated organizations.

The purchase by SPARC-member libraries of new titles published under the banner of SPARC means that the participating library is purchasing more journals; this practice has given rise to some criticism by librarians in that they were already purchasing similar titles. Librarians have historically opposed the proliferation of new journal publishing, seeing it as

creating further inroads on their beleaguered budgets and providing ever increasing revenues to publishers. Although superficially correct, this criticism
fails to recognize the extraordinary achievement of SPARC in fostering alternative forms of publishing to encourage competition with existing costly
commercial publications. SPARC has introduced true competition and
proposed alternative solutions to the high-priced commercial model and in
doing so has helped to rein in the costs of existing titles through providing
some competition.

In 2002, SPARC Europe was founded, representing a strategic alliance
of European research libraries, library organizations, and research institutions. Like its senior partner, SPARC Europe has joined with the Joint Information Systems Committee (JISC) and the Society of College, National
and University Libraries (SCONUL) in the United Kingdom; the Netherlands Cooperative of Research Libraries; and LIBER, the European academic library association. Under the leadership of David Prosser, SPARC
Europe has launched initiatives similar to those of its American counterpart
but with a European focus.[11] Its European base has made SPARC Europe
active in a number of government inquiries on scientific publishing, most
significantly the work of the United Kingdom Government and House of
Commons Science and Technology Committee. SPARC Europe actively
supports the proposed open-access policy of the Research Councils of the
United Kingdom that requires deposit of research into open-access
archives.

PROMOTING PUBLIC ACCESS AT THE
NATIONAL INSTITUTES OF HEALTH AND
THE U.S. NATIONAL LIBRARY OF MEDICINE

With the development of strong and reliable networks and the conversion
of traditional print journals to electronic form, the research community was
beginning to pose questions regarding access, ownership, and costs of the
scientific literature.[12] Librarians responsible for the delivery of scientific and
medical literature to users had been discussing these issues for some time
and welcomed these initiatives from the scientific community. They received strong support in their efforts to provide access to medical information at the turn of the millennium, as the result of initiatives at the U.S. National Institutes of Health and the National Library of Medicine. With an
annual investment in research of more than thirty billion dollars per year,
the National Institutes of Health were concerned with maximizing the

benefits of this funded research by making the published results available as broadly as possible. For its part, the National Library of Medicine was concerned equally with access and the need for a secure and permanent archive of these results. There was a worry that publishers could remove data from their websites. PubMed and PubMed Central placed powerful tools in the hands of librarians and their users. PubMed provided

> a database of citations and abstracts for millions of articles from thousands of journals. It includes links to full-text articles at several thousand journal web sites as well as most of the articles in PubMed Central. PubMed Central (PMC) is an electronic archive of full-text journals offering free access to its contents. PMC contains a few hundred thousand articles, most of which have a corresponding entry in PubMed.[13]

PubMed was developed by the National Center for Biotechnology Information (NCBI) as the host of MEDLINE. It introduced a feature that promoted the tracking of related papers, including pre-MEDLINE data and links to full-text articles appearing in peer-reviewed journals. At the initiation of this program, some seven hundred journal publishers had agreed to participate in this access program.

In 1999, under the leadership of Harold Varmus, the U.S. National Institutes of Health had issued a challenge in the form of a proposal designed to make freely available over the Internet the literature of the life sciences, including biology, medicine, and plant and agricultural science.[14] The National Institutes of Health proposal was to establish a Web-based repository for universal access to the biomedical literature that will be deposited there. Varmus clearly foresaw that this new form of access would alter the economic model of scientific journal publishing from reader/library pays to author pays and stipulated that NIH grant holders could use these funds to support submission and documentation costs associated with depositing in PubMed Central, just as these funds were traditionally used for page and reprint charges by grant holders. From the beginning, the intent was to work with publishers to make the information in PubMed Central available in as rapid and transparent a fashion as possible. The goals of this innovation in the availability of biomedical information were access and a reliable permanent archive of federally funded research activity, goals that would be readily seen by medical librarians as supporting their core values as well. PubMed Central was truly access without borders at the international level. Inaugurated in February 2000 using content from the *Proceedings of the National Academy of Sciences* and *Molecular Biology of the Cell*, it demonstrated the possibility of open access to the medical literature at an early stage, a good ten months prior to the Budapest meeting that produced the Budapest Open Access Initiative. A digital archive of peer-reviewed full-text research reports and electronic journal articles became available globally to anyone with an Internet connection.

A PubMed Central National Advisory Committee under the chairmanship of Nobel laureate Joshua Lederberg was established and included Harold Varmus, now the former director of the National Institutes of Health, who as director had initiated the program to improve access to the medical literature a few years earlier; Paul Ginsparg, who had developed the Los Alamos preprint project in high-energy physics that is today housed at Cornell University; a medical librarian, Michael Homan, from the Mayo Clinic and then president of the Medical Library Association; James Neal from Johns Hopkins and now at Columbia; Jim Williams from the University of Colorado; and Donald Lindberg and other members of the National Library of Medicine. Also included were representatives from the scientific editing and publishing worlds. This well-constituted committee provided breadth of consultation and strength of purpose, laying the groundwork for the continuing development of an essential resource for medical librarians worldwide.

It is not difficult from today's vantage point to imagine the agenda and discussions at these meetings. In fact no imagination is necessary since the full record of those meetings is freely available on the Web. The purpose of PubMed Central and its National Advisory Committee demonstrates the continuing commitment to providing information to all who need it:

> Since the mission of NIH is to conduct and support medical research and to disseminate the results of that research widely to the public and the scientific community, it will make use of electronic publishing technology to fulfill this role by establishing and maintaining PubMed Central.[15]

What is exciting still in retrospect is the fact that at least some appropriate compromises could be reached between the various interest groups represented on the advisory committee to allow this enormous step forward in providing direct access to segments of the medical and scientific literature to all who needed it. The moment was propitious; the technological capabilities existed to house and make available this important medical archive. The goals of the program were ambitious and far-reaching: to create a repository of full-text life sciences research articles that is available to all and to provide a robust digital archive where content not limited to the traditional journal article would be available in new ways.[16]

Vigorous debate arose from the PubMed Central initiative. Both the Varmus initiative at the National Institutes of Health and the Public Library of Science petition signed by thirty thousand scientists had failed to reach the desired result of open accessibility to the literature of science and medicine. The validity of the idea of open access required both further refinement and a galvanizing statement if open access was to emerge as a viable alternative. As described in chapter 10, the Budapest meeting in December 2001 stands at a watershed point in fixing the concept of open access. Emerging here as well is the clearly defined alternative of a new form of publishing. No longer is the discussion focused upon reclaiming the rights of access from the publisher but shifts to a new form of publishing, unfettered by the constraints of commercial ownership.

A one-day meeting was convened by the Howard Hughes Medical Institute, Chevy Chase, Maryland, in April 2003 to stimulate discussion within the biomedical research community regarding how best to ensure as rapidly as possible access to the primary literature of science and medicine. The objective of promoting public access was clear from the beginning, and the participants were invited to create strategies to realize them. Two important considerations were part of the conditions in discussing the objective: open access was to be applied to individual works, not to journals or publishers, and "community standards rather than copyright law" were identified as the means to ensure responsible attribution of published work.[17] The result was the *Bethesda Statement on Open Access Publishing*, released in June 2003, which endorsed open access, recognized that the costs of publishing were an integral part of the research process, urged scientific societies to support open access by encouraging society members to publish in open-access journals, advocated for the tenure process to consider the quality of the article rather than the journal in which it was published, and called on scientists and their societies to engage in educating their colleagues to move toward open access. It is not surprising to find many names already familiar to open-access initiatives engaged in this meeting: Patrick O. Brown and Michael Eisen from the Public Library of Science; Richard Johnson from SPARC; Harold E. Varmus, now president of Memorial Sloan–Kettering Cancer Center; and Jan Velterop, publisher of BioMed Central, to name only a few, as well as Linda Watson, director of the Claude Moore Health Sciences Library, University of Virginia Health System.

A remarkable convergence of influences on access to medical and scientific information was taking place: the profit-centered economic model of commercial journal publishing was increasingly restricting access to medical information to those who could buy it; the conversion of the medical journal from print to electronic form was virtually complete; and the public was demanding access to the results of research for which their tax dollars had paid. Commercial science publishing restricts public access in several ways: through the licensing agreements that restrict libraries in providing access to users not identified under the licensing agreements, and through the high and often prohibitive costs of these licensing agreements. Concerned about both these issues, the U.S. Congress requested that the U.S. National Library of Medicine investigate the rising costs of journal licensing agreements and, in the words of the U.S. House Committee on Appropriations, "identify potential remedies to ensure that taxpayer-funded research remains in the public domain and recommended steps to be taken to alleviate restrictions on access."[18] The Zerhouni report that responded to this initiative of the House Committee on Appropriations, *Access to Biomedical Research Information*, had great relevance to major communities: to the publishing industry, to the library community, and to the people of the United States. In the case of the publishing industry, the report documents, yet again, the highly lucrative industry that commercial science publishing has become. Using data from research libraries in Canada and the United States provided by the Association of Research Libraries (ARL), it demonstrates that in seven years (1986–2001) these libraries spent three times more and received 5 percent fewer titles. Further, it identifies journal prices as especially high in medicine and science, with medical journal increases of 43 percent between 1998 and 2002. Although this pricing information provides a vital element of the report, it was by no means new information to librarians who had been stalwart throughout this period of inflationary increases in providing current published medical information to health professionals and consumers of health care. The report reviews a variety of efforts on the part of researchers, scholars, and librarians, beginning with the Budapest Open Access Initiative (2002), to free the scientific record through open access. It is important to note that the impact of alternative methods of making publicly funded research available, like the high cost of commercial publishing, was a major factor in the resulting recommendations of the NLM report.

This report identifies a variety of motives on the part of medical and scientific publishers. It distinguishes between the "information as commodity" approach, referred to earlier in this book, and the desire to communicate research results to a professional community. It also recognizes the two essential attributes of medical information in the public good: availability, immediate accessibility free of charge; and permanence, secure and perpetual availability in a public repository. It builds upon earlier work to secure current medical information into the future through PubMed Central.[19] Finally, the report challenges the prestige factor of journal titles by affirming the policy of the National Institutes of Health that grants from a major research-funding agency be awarded on the basis of the quality of the research and not in consideration of the particular journal in which results are published.

The report reaffirmed the fundamental social value or public good that is achieved through sharing openly the research results of federally supported biomedical research. It also recognized that scholarly communication in the form of a system of publication that has evolved over three and a half centuries was in a period of profound change. The current economic and legal models needed to be reconceptualized in this new era of public accessibility. In a quintessentially optimistic approach, the report stated that "many publishers will adapt by embracing the opportunity to develop new strategies and services."[20] Future actions recommended are built upon the recognized, reliable, and universally available MEDLINE database, which should include quality journals published in open access, and the continuing development of PubMed Central to provide free access to the public over the Internet. Other actions endorse the use of grant funds to support publication costs in open-access journals, and the recognition of the value of open-access journals.

Reaction to Zerhouni's *Access to Biomedical Research Information* was not slow in coming. In a letter dated August 23, 2004, to Zerhouni and signed by a number of scientific association publishers—the American Institute of Physics, the American Medical Publishers Association, and the American Physiological Society—this segment of the publishing world reacted to a "radical new policy with respect to the publication of NIH funded research."[21] The letter articulates what came to be known as the DC Principles, described in the letter as "an attempt to articulate a compromise between those who advocate immediate and unfettered online access to medical and scientific findings and advocates of the established journal publishing system." The DC Principles assert that the public's right to scientific research is not hampered by the established system of scientific publishing. The letter is a carefully crafted response to the initiatives contained in Zerhouni's report and questions the involvement of government in scientific publishing, a central and government-sponsored repository (PubMed Central), and the provision of worldwide access to research funded by the U.S. taxpayer. It perceives a threat to the integrity of the scientific literature in alternative methods of scientific publishing. Clearly, lines were being drawn in the debate.

The U.S. Congress continued to express concern with insufficient public access to federally funded research and with the costs and limited availability of licensed electronic medical journals. At the heart of the matter was the issue of the right of citizens in the United States to access information for which their tax dollars had paid. Vigorous efforts on behalf of public access to the results of published research funded directly by NIH granting agencies continued. In September 2004, the Appropriations Committee of the U.S. House of Representatives endorsed a proposal to make the complete texts of NIH-funded research available free of charge on PubMed Central. It further recommended that NIH develop a policy that required the deposit of an electronic copy of any manuscript supported by NIH funding in PubMed Central upon the acceptance of the article in the directory of PubMed. Mandating deposit created further opposition within the publishing community, and following considerable consultation and lobbying, the language of this directive was modified in February 2005. The National Institutes of Health issued its "Policy on Enhancing Public Access to Archived Publications Resulting from NIH-Funded Research." Submission of articles to PubMed Central was to begin on May 2, 2005, but it was merely requested, not required. Submission timing was changed to as soon as possible or within twelve months. When Elias Zerhouni, director of the National Institutes of Health, made the decision to make deposit of the published results of NIH-funded research voluntary, the *Washington Post* reported the decision as "a compromise between competing forces that had lobbied the agency intensely."[22] Zerhouni saw this more permissive, gentler approach as an encouragement to the research community to make its published work publicly available. He saw the NIH policy on public access as fundamental to changing scientific publishing by "opening up a venue for scientists to do the right thing" and went on to assert that "the goal is to make this research available to the public without damaging the peer review process."[23] Doubtlessly, this more permissive language pleased many publishers, especially as it allowed a firewall to continue to protect restricted access to the most recently published results.

Advocates of transparency and public accessibility criticized the decision and foresaw a manipulation of the process whereby publishers might urge slow public release of the research, subverting the NIH intent. Voluntary deposit gave ample opportunity to impede the system. It is not surprising, then, that efforts to push forward broader public access had to continue. SPARC recommended that the NIH report to the public and

Congress on the number of articles that were being deposited in PubMed Central.[24] In June 2005, the U.S. House Appropriations Committee again expressed concern that the goal of timely public access to the published result of NIH-funded research might not be being achieved under the present permissive system, and requested that a progress report on the success of requesting researchers to deposit their published research results in PubMed Central be prepared.[25] In October 2005, in response to the NIH policy statement, a proposal was made by fifty-seven medical and scientific nonprofit publishers in the United States to the U.S. National Institutes of Health to assist NIH in enhancing free public access. The proposal involved linking the articles on these publishers' websites to the listings in MEDLINE, and was designed to help NIH in its efforts to offer public access to the results of research that had been funded by NIH. This voluntary program was designed to guarantee that only the final official published version of the article was available, eliminating public anxiety regarding the presence of serious errors in earlier versions of articles.

The story is far from over. In December 2005 the question of open access was again an issue, this time on the floor of the U.S. Senate, when a bill was introduced by Senator Joseph Lieberman to mandate open access to research results, based on public funding. This bill, known as the "CURES Act," also calls for a new department within the National Institutes of Health that would have as its mandate the transfer of research into therapy. The act applies to the final peer-reviewed manuscript of the author, which must be submitted to PubMed Central within four months of its publication. The bill is likely to be strongly argued, since it not only shortens the timeframe for submission but also returns to the earlier and stronger language of mandating as opposed to requesting.

FURTHER INITIATIVES ON
BEHALF OF PUBLIC SCIENCE: PLoS

Public accessibility of medical and scientific research results may advance in several ways. In the case of PubMed Central it advances by making certain that the established system of scholarly communication feeds a central and publicly accessible repository. Here the existing publishing system is used to meet the public need. The existing system is being reengineered, and the debate is about whether it is being too radically reengineered. A more fundamental change occurs when a new system of publishing is adopted; one that is rooted in open access and shifts the economic model from reader or library pays to author pays. This model was boldly advanced with the launching in October 2003 of the first in a series of journals in the Public Library of Science series, *PLoS Biology*. On the board of directors of this initiative is Harold Varmus, so familiar through the initiatives he attempted while director of NIH; Patrick O. Brown; Michael Eisen, who had been at the Budapest meeting; Paul Ginsparg; Laurence Lessig; and the librarian Beth Weil, from the Marian Koshland Bioscience and Natural Resources Library, University of California at Berkeley. From the earliest moment, the board was determined to produce a journal that met the highest possible standard of peer review and at the same time one that would be freely and publicly available. The maintenance of quality was critical, since the threat to the sacred idea of peer review was an argument frequently used as one of the most compelling reasons for maintaining the existing commercially dominated model of scientific publishing. *PLoS Biology* was available in a high-quality print edition, designed to emphasize its permanence and excellence. It was simultaneously available freely over the Internet to be read anywhere by anyone and used in any way as long as there was appropriate recognition of the source of the information. In introducing this new journal, Harold Varmus stated that

> Scientists want their work to be seen and used. The outstanding science in the first issue of PLoS Biology shows that many scientists believe in open access and are willing to demonstrate their convictions by sending their best work to a brand-new and non-traditional journal.[26]

Patrick O. Brown, also a member of the Board of Directors of PLoS, was equally enthusiastic about this new journal:

> Science thrives on the free flow of information. By removing restrictions on the sharing of knowledge—assuring that anyone, anywhere can access the latest research findings—PloS will speed the pace of scientific discovery.[27]

The first impact factor for *PLoS Biology* assessed by the Institute for Scientific Information was 13.9, which placed this journal among the most cited. This was an unusual result, since the journal was less than two years old at the time of assessment and from an "alternative" publisher. The assessment was based on citations in 2004 to articles that appeared in 2003.[28]

In October 2004, *PLoS Medicine* was launched, described by the editors as "a medical journal for the Internet Age." Like *PLoS Biology*, its aim was to unlock the literature, making it available immediately and freely to the public worldwide. It maintains the founding principles of the Public Library of Science including the importance of high-quality submissions. "The revolutionary idea of anyone being able to read any article is possible"[29] was an important part of the launch of this new journal. It uses the Creative Commons Attribution License for content licensing. The importance of this approach to copyright for open access is explored in the following chapter on copyright.

EUROPEAN INITIATIVES FOR CHANGE

In October 2003, a Conference on Open Access to Knowledge in the Sciences and Humanities was convened at the Max Planck Institute in Berlin resulting in the Berlin Declaration. The conference attendees asserted their agreement with the spirit of both the Budapest Open Access Initiative and the Bethesda Statement on Open Access. Participants were committed to advancing the communication of medical and scientific research results worldwide over the Internet. The Berlin Declaration recognized that "in order to realize the vision of a global and accessible representation of knowledge, the future Web has to be sustainable, interactive, and transparent. Content and software tools must be openly accessible and compatible."[30] The Berlin Declaration considered open access not only to the published literature but also to raw research data and metadata, digital representations of pictorial and graphic materials, and multimedia. It supports "free, irrevocable worldwide right of access to and license to copy, use, distribute, transmit and display publicly" and the deposit of a complete version of an article in at least one online repository that promotes open access without restriction, long-term archiving, and interoperability. Coming at this particular point in the growing understanding of the meaning of open access, the Berlin Declaration considers the full range of issues involved in providing public access worldwide to the scientific literature. It builds upon earlier initiatives such as BOAI to provide a rich and complete position statement. The need to transform the legal and financial framework of scientific publishing to realize the universal goal of open access is clearly and strongly expressed.

Given the international nature of research in science and medicine, it is not surprising to find similar initiatives and debate regarding change in the existing system of scholarly communication in the United Kingdom. In June 2005, the Research Councils of the United Kingdom (RCUK) proposed mandatory deposit of papers resulting from research funded by the Councils. The Research Councils include councils serving all disciplines—arts and humanities, the social sciences, science, engineering, and medicine. The proposal required deposit of articles in an e-print repository, either institutional or subject based, "at the earliest opportunity."[31] The policy was to apply only to newly funded research, that is, research funded since October 1, 2005. Authors of articles resulting from grants awarded before October 1, 2005, would be encouraged but not required to deposit their articles. RCUK recognized the transformative nature of information technology evident in electronic publishing and open-access journals, and grant applicants were encouraged to include in their submissions for funding the costs associated with author-pays journals. The Joint Information Systems Committee (JISC) and the Research Libraries Network (RLN) supported this RCUK public-access initiative as a matter of principle. As of March, 2005, a total of fifty open-access repositories existed in the United Kingdom and the librarian community became proactive in facilitating the deposit of articles.[32]

OPENING ACCESS IN THE DEVELOPING WORLD

Scientific communication between the developed and the developing world faces two serious challenges: how scientists worldwide can have better access to the literature created by the developing world, and how the developing world can acquire improved access to the literature of the developed world. Each of these challenges presents a unique set of biases and problems.

Providing access to the literature of medicine that is created by researchers in the developing world has not historically been seen as a serious problem until recent years. Indeed, there may still remain sectors of the scientific community that question the need to address this issue. There are some legitimate reasons for this: medical researchers face today extraordinary challenges in keeping up with the vast amount of relevant published literature that already exists. Adding to this plethora of information may not be viewed as helpful to the scientist whose information awareness services are already overloaded. However, in the arena of clinical medicine, there is now a much fuller understanding of the importance of knowing the literature in clinical medicine and epidemiology in the developing world. The twentieth century has provided ample evidence of the importance of international health. The pandemic flu of 1917 was perhaps a wake-up call, but other political issues—war and recovery—and a less well-developed global communication system inhibited the development of a growing consciousness of the importance of the issue of developing-world science. The outbreak of AIDS in the early 1980s brought with it a fuller and fearful understanding of the implications of the international transmission of disease. Immigration and public health laws in many developed countries dated from the first part of the twentieth century and prevented the immigration of people who suffered from diseases such as tuberculosis, diseases that by the end of the last century were largely under control. New legislation was needed for new diseases. But what if those diseases were not yet named? And what if those diseases were incubating but not able to be detected by screening? It had become clear by the last quarter of the twentieth century that communicable diseases and their irradiation could no longer be treated as a national issue, if only for reasons of enlightened self-interest.

In the context of an enriched understanding of the need to improve the awareness of disease and its treatment in the developing world, the literature of the countries of the Southern Hemisphere needs to be reviewed and better understood in the countries of the North. How this can best be accomplished was not clear at first, given the strong and escalating emphasis on critical referring and quality assurance in all the standard access services used by the medical community. The rigorous selection process for inclusion of a journal in the MEDLINE database, for example, could not be readily expanded without influencing the selection criteria and goals of the program. Including a fuller representation of developing-world medical publishing in the search and retrieval systems of the literature of developed countries was not a viable way of providing improved exposure to this literature.

Extraordinary progress in accessing the literature of Latin American countries is being made through Scientific Electronic Library Online (Sci-ELO).[33] SciELO was designed to overcome the barriers in the distribution and dissemination that arise in the developing world and limit the use of indigenous scientific information. It provides a platform for the electronic publishing of Latin American scientific journals of contributing countries over the Internet, a necessary adjunct to the access tools of North America, considering that fewer than sixty out of the perhaps fifteen hundred titles that originate in Latin America are included in the MEDLINE database. SciELO recognized the importance of capturing this information for reasons of public policy development and economic and social development, even if all of the medical content did not meet the criteria used by the major international information services. This remarkable program is the result of collaboration between the government of Brazil, BIREME, the Latin America Center on Health Sciences Information, the Pan American Health Organization, and scientific journal editors. Since its beginnings in 1998, SciELO has been engaged in the use and evaluation of electronic scientific publishing on the Internet. SciELO has dynamic links to MEDLINE and creates a portal to provide access to multiple sites in the Spanish- and Portuguese-speaking worlds. One particularly successful journal, the *Brazilian Journal of Medical and Biological Research*, is available in open access in SciELO; it is also indexed in ISI, BIOSIS, PsychInfo, and MEDLINE. Since it became available in open access in SciELO, citations to the journal have increased from 895 in 1997 to 2,043 in 2005. The editor of the journal believes that "open access can have a significant positive effect on journals published in developing countries by making them available to the world. However, not all journals will benefit. This will depend on the quality and content of the journal."[34]

SciELO provides a powerful demonstration of the value of the open-access publishing model in the developing world. In evaluating the model, it is relevant to note that the relative poverty of Brazilian libraries makes the subscription model, where the library pays, less desirable. Yet in this case, poverty has become, if not a virtue, at least something of an asset, since the lower costs of open-access publishing have given the journal much broader circulation and citability.

Using open access to publish and promote the science of the developing world provides an organized and viable solution to accessing the science of a country, both nationally and internationally. But the developing world must also have access to the scientific literature created in the developed world. Neither of the two best-known current systems that are working to meet this need are models of open access but use alternative funding models to attempt to meet this need. These two quite distinct systems are Electronic Information for Libraries (eIFL)[35] and Health Internetwork Access to Research Initiative (HINARI),[36] a cooperative venture between the World Health Organization and commercial publishing.

Electronic Information for Libraries is supported in part by the Information Program of the Open Society Institute. While it is closely linked with the Open Access Program of OSI, eIFL is a purchasing consortium that buys large amounts of electronic journals from publishers for a multinational membership. It is focused on transition countries, especially the countries of the former Soviet Union, but also includes many African and Asian counties. Started in 1999 as a joint initiative of the Open Society Institute and EBSCO, it has membership in fifty countries and supports consortium building in the fullest sense of the word, through the promotion of numerous workshops that train information professionals on a wide number of topics. Regular meetings of a broadly representative board allow for feedback, exchange, and modification of the programs to meet the needs of participating countries. Because of the strong link to the Open Access Program of the Open Society Institute, it promotes open-access publishing while at the same time acquiring toll-gated information for the benefit of its members. Perhaps this fact, more than anything we have discussed, illustrates the transition through which libraries worldwide are passing.

HINARI was conceived to provide access in the developing world to a large collection of commercially published biomedical and health journals. Almost three thousand journal titles are available in online version only to more than one hundred countries that qualify, based on a GNP per capita of less than $1,000 according to figures provided by the World Bank. Countries whose GNP is between $1,000 and $3,000 pay $1,000 per year per institution. A reduced number of titles are provided free of charge to those institutions that are in the second category but are unable to pay the $1,000 annual access fee. This collaboration between commercial publishers promises much, if one assumes that the necessary information infrastructure for electronic access is available and that a degree of health information literacy is present "on the ground" to ensure that the information is accessed. Clearly, providing electronic-only access (and the program makes no provision for print) in a undeveloped information environment is not likely to derive the kinds of benefits that access to high-quality medical information should provide. Connectivity and training to say nothing of reliable sources of electricity are indispensable adjuncts to effective use of health information at a grassroots level, and this has been demonstrated repeatedly in developed as well as developing countries. An evaluation of the program some five years following its announcement would be most interesting.

As this drama of accessibility and public rights continues within the United States, similar issues are being argued over around the globe. The next steps will be important to medical librarians throughout the world. If merely recommending deposit of articles has not provided the desired results, will more stringent legal requirements be placed on authors? If so, will copyright be used to restrict deposit, thereby protecting commercial publishing interests? As publishers discuss with authors the deposit of their articles in PubMed Central in the United States or in institutional and subject repositories elsewhere, will they insist on ever increasing extension of the required time of deposit from one to two or three years? Will the idea of a publicly accessible, permanent archive of publications resulting from government-funded research be allowed to wither because of publishers' control of copyright? Will authors be encouraged to take back their rights to the results of their published works? Librarians have a key role to play in two areas: in helping authors better to understand the restraints of copyright, and in facilitating the transfer of documents to openly accessible repositories. Central to the question of deposit in open-access repositories is making the process as straightforward and simple as possible. This suggests an important direction not only for medical librarians but for all librarians. In providing access to scientific information, the library will not be limited to acting as the conduit for licensed information for content on remote proprietary servers. The proactive promotion of new forms of public access to the published literature and to new kinds of information such as large data files and other research information on which published research results were founded is part of the legitimate mandate of the medical information specialist.

NOTES

1. David A. Kronick, *A History of Scientific and Technical Periodicals*, 2d ed. (Metuchen, NJ: Scarecrow Press, 1976), 34.

2. Jean-Claude Guedon, *In Oldenburg's Long Shadow—Librarians, Research Scientists, Publishers and the Control of Scientific Publishing* (Washington, DC: Association of Research Libraries, 2001), 5.

3. Kronick, *History of Scientific and Technical Periodicals*, 37.

4. Kronick, *History of Scientific and Technical Periodicals*, 78.

5. Derek de Sola Price, *Little Science, Big Science* (New York: Columbia University Press, 1963).

6. OECD Working Party on the Information Economy, *Digital Broadband Content: Scientific Publishing* (Paris: OECD, 2005): 30.

7. A. J. Meadows, ed., *Development of Science Publishing in Europe* (Amsterdam: Elsevier Science, 1980), viii.

8. Meadows, *Development of Science Publishing*, 249.

9. See http://www.arl.org/arl/proceedings/130/bus.mtg.html (accessed August 16, 2005).

10. See http://www.arl.org/sparc/about/index.html (accessed July15, 2006).

11. See http://www.sparceurope.org (accessed August 25, 2005).

12. Two articles that represent particularly well the nature of this questioning are Steven Bachrach et al., "Who Should Own Scientific Papers?" *Science* 281, no. 5382 (September 1998), 1459–60; and Barry P. Markovitz, "Biomedicine's Electronic Publishing Paradigm Shift: Copyright Policy and PubMed Central," *Journal of the American Medical Informatics Assn.* 7, no. 3 (May–June 2000): 222–29.

13. See http://www.pubmedcentral.nih.gov/about/faq.html (accessed August 24, 2005). This site provides a wealth of current information on developments of these services.

14. See http://www.nih.gov/welcome/director/ebiomed/ebi.htm (accessed August 23, 2005).

15. U.S. Department of Health and Human Services, National Institutes of Health, National Library of Medicine, National Center for Biotechnology Information, Summary Minutes of the Meeting of April 28, 2005, 1.

16. A description of the beginnings of this work is contained in Michael Homan's address to the Medical Library Association. See *Bulletin of the Medical Library Association* 89, no. 1 (January 2001): 120.

17. "Bethesda Statement on Open Access Publishing," released June 20, 2003. http://www.earlham.edu/~peters/fos/bethesda.htm (accessed December 12, 2005).

18. Elias A. Zerhouni, *Access to Biomedical Research Information* (Washington, DC: U.S. National Library of Medicine May 2004), 1.

19. PubMed Central is a digital archive/repository of articles from 130 journals in biomedicine. It was established by the U.S. National Library of Medicine in 2000.

20. Zerhouni, *Access to Biomedical Research Information*, 11.

21. Letter to Zerhouni, www.dcprinciples.org/zerhouni.pdf (accessed December 8, 2005).

22. *Washington Post*, February 4, 2005, cited at http://www.medicalnewstoday.com/medicalnews.php?newsid=19675 (accessed August 25, 2005).

23. *Chicago Tribune*, February 4, 2005, http://wwwmedicalnewstoday.com/medicalnews.php?newsid=19675 (accessed August 25, 2005).

24. SPARC, "The NIH Public Access Policy," http://www.arl.org/sparc/author/index.html (accessed March 31, 2005).

25. An excellent summary of developments to this point was presented by Sheldon Kotzin at an IFLA Preconference Workshop on Open Access in Oslo August 13, 2005. He described the contents of PubMed Central as of May 2005 as 385,000 items from 187 journals with more than 50 percent from digitized back issues.

26. Quoted in PLoS Public Library of Science, "Public Library of Science Launches *PLoS Biology*: New Open-Access Journal Will Increase Access to Scientific Research and Speed Scientific Discovery," http://www.plos.org/news/announce_pbiolaunch.html (accessed November 30, 2005).

27. See http://www/plos.org/news/announce_pbiolaunch.html (accessed November 30, 2005).

28. "The First Impact Factor of PLoS Biology—13.9," liblicense-l@lists.yale.edu (Rebecca Kennison, June 23, 2005).

29. "Prescription for a Healthy Journal: Take Monthly, at No Cost; Reaches Six Billion," http://medicine.plosjournals.org/perlserv/?request=getdocument&doi=10.1371/journal.pmed.0010022 (accessed December 10, 2005).

30. Berlin   Declaration,   http://www.zim.mpg.de/openaccess-berlin/ berlindeclaration.html (accessed December 14, 2005).

31. Research Councils UK, "RCUK Announces Proposed Position on Access to Research Outputs," news release, June 28, 2005, http://www.rcuk.ac.uk/press/ 20050628openaccess.asp (accessed September 17, 2005).

32. See especially a brochure prepared by JISC at http://www.jisc.ac.uk/ uploaded-documents/QandA-Doc-final.pdf (accessed December 11, 2005).

33. See http://wwwscielo.org/model_en.htm (accessed September 7, 2005).

34. Lewis Joel Greene, "Effect of Open Access on a Scientific Journal Published in a Developing Country" (paper presented at the 9th World Congress on Health Information and Libraries, International Seminar on Open Access, Salvador de Bahia, Brazil, September 23, 2005).

35. See http://www.eifl.net/ (accessed October 1, 2005).

36. See http://www.who.int/hinari/en/ (accessed October 1, 2005).

12

CONTROLLING COPYRIGHT:
THE NECESSARY BALANCE

An appropriate balance between the rights of creators and those of users of copyrighted material has been the continuing goal of enlightened copyright legislation. The arrival of the Internet and the World Wide Web with server/browser capability to provide unparalleled amounts of content has threatened this balance. Such a statement is ironic in that the development of the Internet was based on openness and an overwhelming desire to build a worldwide system of communication. Who controls Internet content and who can access that content has become a question of great significance in all aspects of life.

In many nations of the North, the rights of the library to provide access to copyrighted material were enshrined in the concepts of "fair use" or "fair dealing" and the idea of the rights of "first sale." The right of first sale restricts the rights of copyright holders in the control and distribution of their work by asserting that once a work has been sold, the right of a copyright holder to control further distribution ends. Given this protection, the library should, in principle, be free to provide access to the information that it has acquired to whomever it wishes. Fair use and first sale rights combine to form, at least in theory, powerful protection by legislation to guarantee access to information for the public good. The preservation of and access to the accumulated wisdom of the past are of equal importance in society. As copyright expires on works, they become part of the public domain and may be considered as "public goods," forming a rich historical basis for the creation of new works. Fair use, rights of first sale, limited-term copyright, and other guidelines have been developed to ensure access to information and the preservation of the balance between the rights of users and of creators. The length of time that a work remains under copyright varies considerably between countries. However, the essential point is that it is a form of protection that is limited by time. The more that limitation period is extended, the greater the erosion of the public interest.

As systems of scholarly communication converted from print to electronic form, enormous shifts in how new knowledge was communicated occurred. The practicing members of the scientific and medical research communities were fully engaged in the application of new technologies in their research. Further, they were highly sophisticated in using networks to communicate data and research findings to each other and, when that research was ready for publication, to their publishers. Publishers introduced software to facilitate the submission and review of manuscripts, and journal production was even further improved. These important developments and the speed of scientific progress itself did not give researchers much time to ponder the issues surrounding copyright. Signing the traditional copyright release form provided by publishers was not an issue for deep reflection.

Signing deals with publishers for large chunks of science journals, including clauses that restricted access, became second nature to many librarians, as we have described in earlier chapters. Simply put, high-quality content was key, and toll-gated content was highly profitable. Publishers, after all, had to ensure that more than one copy of a journal set was purchased, and in theory, given the development of telecommunications, only one copy was necessary, provided there were no restrictions on access. Contract law gradually came to replace "fair use," or "fair dealing," as it is known in Canada. This was equally true in deals with publishers involving millions of dollars and in agreements regarding CD-ROMs with their shrink-wrap licenses. Access to information in the electronic world clearly needed new legislation to cover the radically altered ways in which content was being delivered. All content—music, scholarly information, movies, government information—needed to be considered.

In chapter 1, we discussed the "tragedy of the commons" as described by Hardin and argued that information, especially information that resulted from taxpayer dollars, should be considered as "public goods." In his lucid analysis of this question, Larry Lessig defines public goods as those resources that are accessible without the permission of someone else.[1] They are resources held in common, and he includes as part of his definition the distinction previously mentioned between those resources that are consumed by being used and those that are not. However, this definition does not fully satisfy, and he argues further that resources must be defined by their characteristics and how the particular resource relates to the community. Unlike resources in nature, there must be sufficient benefit in the production of man-made resources that will ensure their continuing production. The appropriate balance between creator and consumer of material in the commons, as seen by Lessig, is a useful window from which to view the issues surrounding copyright in a digital era.

FAIR USE ENSHRINED

In the case of *Williams & Wilkins v. U.S. National Library of Medicine* (see chapter 5, pp. 90–91) what was regarded as "fair use" in practice was not necessarily "fair use" in the eyes of a publisher. But this dispute was not only a clash over the interpretation of fair use between the user and the creator, in this case the publisher. It marked the beginning of attempts to resolve border disputes that arose as new technologies were being introduced in the delivery of information. Recall that this case evolved from a dispute over photocopying practices. Today digital "copying" creates possibilities far beyond photocopying. But the case remains an important landmark for libraries in their efforts to provide access to information to all who need it. The fact that the publisher launched a suit against a public institution rather than the private sector, in which similar practices also existed, has proven significant. As one communications scholar has put it,

> Williams & Wilkins attacked public appropriation of copyrighted works in order to preserve the integrity of its copyrights. By making the public sector appear parasitical, the suit obscured the fact that vast amounts of scientific research and information are produced and made available due to public funding.[2]

In finding that the copying of materials at the National Library of Medicine was justified and within the law under the provision of fair use, the Court of Claims concluded that the claimant had not been hurt by these practices of the National Library of Medicine in providing photocopies of journal articles in Williams & Wilkins journals. More important for the future of the distribution of medical information, jurors found that the practice of medicine would be harmed if the distribution of this information was curtailed. Martin Cummings, director of the National Library of Medicine at the time, clearly appreciated how much was at stake in this case. It is also important that these legal decisions regarding the public interest and the right of the library to make copyrighted material available to those who needed it had been confirmed prior to the writing of new legislation that codified the practice of fair use.

In 1976 important revisions to the U.S. Copyright Act appeared that provided precise definitions for fair use, ones that the medical library community could work with at an operational level in fulfilling their core responsibilities of providing access to medical information for all who need to use it. Medical librarians reacted positively to the record keeping required of them under these new guidelines—after some initial grumbling, probably justified by the burden of having to prove compliance if required. These efforts have been documented in the pages of the *Journal of the Medical Library Association*.[3]

THE U.S. DIGITAL MILLENNIUM COPYRIGHT ACT

The need to revisit copyright legislation in the digital era gave birth in the United States to the Digital Millennium Copyright Act (DMCA) in 1998. With the proverbial wisdom of hindsight, it is easy to understand the problems created by DMCA and to appreciate that the act has since suffered from unforeseen developments. In retrospect, the medical adage of "do no harm" might have been helpful, but the various interest groups and their polarization gave momentum to the creation of this legislation, the implications of which are still being argued over.

One much-discussed aspect of the DMCA is the prohibition of circumvention techniques and the introduction of anticircumvention regulation. It amends the Copyright Act (Title 17 U.S.C.) by introducing new rights of owners of copyrights and limits the rights of users when copyrighted works are accessed digitally. While introducing anticircumvention regulation, the act did not clarify or define this restriction sufficiently for users "on the ground." Owners of content and young hackers were equally unclear about what constituted effective methods of technological protection. Licensing and contract law appeared virtually to replace the guiding principle of "fair use" in the digital age. It became essential for all interested parties to understand the implications of the DMCA better. There were cases in which the use of antiencryption software was legitimate, and there were also instances of exceptions that needed to be identified in the use of copyrighted material for personal, research, or teaching purposes. Definitive lists of exceptions are dangerous because the expectation is that everything that is not specifically permitted is, by omission, prohibited. Also an issue for librarians was the right of the public to access information that had been open to them in libraries previously when it was in print form.

Clearly, much mopping up had to be done, and the National Research Council (NRC) of the United States commissioned a study by a committee of experts that appeared two years after the passing of the DMCL. The result was *The Digital Dilemma*,[4] a thoughtful analysis of the legal issues arising from computer technology and intellectual property. More was at stake here than the publications of the research community. Valuable scientific databases and other sources of information not found in the traditional literature were becoming available over the Internet, and whether they were to become proprietary was a critical issue. Often caught in the spotlight of the entertainment industry and their issues, legislative vision may have been dimmed to some of the other pressing concerns regarding copyright in the digital era. Yet this criticism is probably unjust inasmuch as the tremendous complexity of each type of intellectual property that required protection was so great that developing the necessary portmanteau legislation to cover all intellectual property was a most difficult task.

With its broad and well-chosen representation, the NRC committee included diverse interest groups and specialists to address controversies in a number of areas. In fact, the work was accomplished by several working groups, a Committee on Intellectual Property Rights and the Emerging Information Infrastructure; a Computer Science and Telecommunications Board; and a Commission on Physical Sciences, Mathematics, and Applications. A number of briefs from a variety of interest groups were presented during the creation of this far-reaching document.

In their work, the committee identified, inter alia, the particular concerns of libraries in relation to copyright in the digital age: archiving and preservation of the public record and cultural heritage materials, the need for a clear understanding of what constitutes "fair use" in the digital era, and the issue of library liability for patrons who violate publishers' copyright on a library network.[5] It is important to note that there exists in this summary of concerns the expectation that fair use will continue to exist, despite the increasing use of contract law in negotiating rights of access between publishers and libraries. There was recognition of the dilemma faced by librarians as they attempted to reach agreements with some publishers to preserve public accessibility of licensed materials. Although concessions regarding "fair use" were welcomed as a pragmatic solution, this was not a guarantee of the preservation of the concept of fair use, nor did it meet the expectations of librarians with regard to fair-use entitlements.

In their conclusions, the authors of *The Digital Dilemma* recognized the importance of securing public access, a goal of copyright that should be independent of the media of communication of the copyrighted material. But they had to grapple with the basic reality that in the print environment a sufficient number of copies of a work would be purchased to guarantee an appropriate balance between the need to compensate creators and publishers and maintaining the public availability of works. In the digital environment, the new reality was that one copy could serve all needs, provided that the technological infrastructure was in place. Their conclusion is a recommendation that

> representatives from government, rights holders, publishers, libraries and other cultural heritage institutions, the public, and technology providers should convene to begin a discussion of models for public access to information that are mutually workable in the context of the widespread use of licensing and technical protection services.[6]

As we all know, "the devil is in the detail." In the interim since these recommendations, now five years old, we have witnessed continuing discussion and debate. More important, we have seen the enormous strengthening of the thrust toward open access and the rise of alternatives to the present situation that uses copyright as a linchpin to guarantee the market share from which large commercial publishers have historically benefited.

A PARALLEL NORTH OF THE BORDER

Like the United States, by the 1990s Canada needed to revisit its copyright legislation, represented by the Canadian Copyright Act of 1985, and for the same reasons: legislation needed to meet the needs of regulation in a digital world. Further, as a signatory to the World Intellectual Property Organization Copyright and Performance and Phonograms Treaties, Canada needed to develop appropriate parallel legislation at the national level to comply with this multinational agreement to which it had committed. As already seen with regard to American libraries, Canadian librarians demonstrated the same concern with protecting the interests of users in any legislation that addressed the rights of creators, users, and third-party providers. Canadian copyright revision took place a few years later than in the United States, but the Canadian experience does not appear to have benefited from the lessons that could have been learned from the U.S. Digital Millennium Copyright Act.

In Canada, responsibility for copyright is shared between two departments of the federal government: Heritage Canada and Industry Canada. Heritage Canada is the cultural arm of the federal bureaucracy, concerned with the arts in Canada, those who create the arts and the protection of their rights. This alone would suggest that the interests of librarians would not be well represented by this branch of government. Industry Canada, as the name suggests, is focused on industry and technology, the transfer of knowledge, and the relationship between the creation of new knowledge and the economy. This split is an interesting one. It mirrors an important dichotomy that must be considered in relation to published works, copyright, and scholarly communication.

Scientists are not motivated to write and publish articles by the promise of direct financial remuneration. While it is true that their publications may result in prestige and career advancement that ultimately provide financial advantages, financial gain is at best an indirect result. Indeed, the broader the distribution of a scientific article, the greater the benefits to the scientist. Copyright protection in this instance might be a detriment. At the other end of the spectrum is the creator of an artistic work whose livelihood may depend upon the royalties that result from it. In this case the protection of copyright legislation is essential to survival. Canada, because of its governmental structure, seems positioned to represent both sets of interests, but this has not been the case. The problem stems from the need for greater granularity in the analysis of "creator" and "user" and the need to recognize the possibility that effective legislation must recognize these differences. The Canadian Parliament received Bill C-60 in its first reading in the House of Commons, June 20, 2005, following years of discussion and review. Subsequent commentary indicates that it has failed to produce the necessary balance as a first principle. The drafters of this revision appear to have been convinced that the need for legal protection must increase directly as the ease with which material may be distributed, and hence copyright legislation in the digital age must provide even greater protection.

Interlibrary loan provision under Canadian copyright legislation is covered in amendments to the copyright act known as C-32 that were passed in 1997.[7] Two copyright collectives, CanCopy for English-speaking Canada and Union des Ecrivaines et Ecrivains Quebecois (UNEQ) for Quebec, exist, and the need for clarification of the rights provided under fair dealing was important. Unfortunately C-32 did not enshrine the concept of fair dealing and provide a degree of assurance that it would be the guiding principle by which libraries would operate. It introduced a series of exceptions under which materials could be copied that would be available for the use of libraries, museums, and archives. Copyright laws provide the basis for decisions in the dispute over rights, and this division between fair dealing and library exceptions was resolved in what is thought of in Canadian and U.S. library circles as a landmark dispute between a legal publisher and the Law Society of Upper Canada.[8] The court upheld the rights of the library, and in its judgment recognized that a library could use the concept of fair dealing in the first instance to prove that it was behaving legally and fairly, resorting to the exceptions provided to libraries only if it were unable to argue that fair dealing applied.[9]

RESTORING THE BALANCE: CREATIVE COMMONS

From the murkiness of encroaching restrictions on the concept of fair use and the insertion or substitution of contract into many aspects of library agreements arose Creative Commons, an organization founded and led by legal experts in cyberlaw and intellectual property. The cleverness of Creative Commons lies in the fact that it encourages the use of licensing to limit the absolute control of a created work by the publisher or producer of that work. In doing so, Creative Commons is working to restore the necessary balance between the rights of authors or owners of a created work. As they state,

> Creative Commons licenses are based on copyright. So it applies to all works that are protected by copyright law. The kinds of works that are protected by copyright law are books, websites, blogs, photographs, films, videos, songs, and other audio and visual recordings, for example. . . . Creative Commons gives you the ability to dictate how others may exercise your copyright rights—such as the right of others to copy your work, make derivative works or adaptations of your work, to distribute your work and/or make money from your work. They do not give you the ability to restrict anything that is otherwise permitted by exceptions or limitations to copyright—including, importantly, fair use or fair dealing—nor do they give you the ability to control anything that is not protected by copyright law, such as facts and ideas.[10]

In its short history since 2001, Creative Commons has provided model licenses to assist authors and other creators who wish to make their work more publicly available. In doing so, it provides creators of copyrighted material with an alternative to the full surrender of rights of ownership to the publisher. It requires authors to determine, a priori, if they have the right to register a previously copyrighted work using a Creative Commons license. It alerts authors to ask themselves how much of their rights they are willing to assign to publishers and to other holders of copyright in order to have a work published and made available.

Creative Commons offers a solution, in part, to the problem of enlarging access to copyrighted work beyond the scope of present restrictions imposed on their distribution. It encourages an increased awareness on the part of authors and other creators of their rights to their own material and its distribution. As such, it is a distinctively different approach from that of the U.S. National Institutes of Health or the Research Councils of the United Kingdom, which require or recommend deposit of publications resulting from research funded by taxpayers in publicly accessible repositories such as PubMed Central. Creative Commons' approach relies on a reinterpretation of creative rights, rather than on the insistence of public rights. Together these approaches provide powerful alternatives to the locking up of information that could support the public good. They restore a more balanced conception of the rights of creators and users of copyrighted materials.

DATABASE PROTECTION AT THE INTERNATIONAL LEVEL: WIPO AND THE PUBLIC GOOD

The U.S. Digital Millennium Copyright Act provoked debate regarding the protection of databases and the use of antiencryption devices. The issues that it addressed were the result of the arrival of the digital age and were being discussed in legislatures in many countries and at the international level. Worldwide copyright issues are governed by agencies of the United Nations, the World Trade Organization (WTO), and the World Intellectual Property Organization (WIPO), which seek to harmonize intellectual property rights across countries.

Strengthening controls on intellectual property and the rights of the creator appears to be in the interests of the developed world, and attempts to tighten and increase these controls is viewed with alarm by the developing world and their advocates. This division is perhaps simplistic and arbitrary, but it serves to characterize the nature of the discourse for the past decade since the Agreement on Trade-Related Aspects of Intellectual Property (TRIPS) was approved in 1995 as part of the General Agreement on Tariff and Trade (GATT). Like the Berne Convention of 1886 that established copyright protection in the print world, this agreement seeks the formal ratification of the signatories in the participating countries. Countries that sign off on the agreement agree to these standards but are free to establish higher standards within their own borders. However, they must observe the standards of protection that are set. Ratification by a county requires thorough debate. In the course of that debate the implications for the public good are being exposed.

It is important to remember that within GATT it was easier to obtain the necessary majority for ratification in those countries that supported greater protection of databases and patents. GATT also allowed effective sanctions against those who did not comply with the new legal measures. Many voices of concern were raised against the impact on the developing world of stronger and more restrictive intellectual property and patent protection.[11] TRIPS was modified in 2001 to allow developing nations to manufacture and use cheap patented drugs in periods of public health crisis, a direct response to the world AIDS epidemic. Later, the 2004 "Development Agenda"[12] pushed WIPO to pay attention to the needs of developing countries in the crafting of policy on intellectual property with an objective of providing more equitable access to knowledge worldwide. These were major achievements and they have kept alive the debate over whether the developing world is better served by strong intellectual property protection, as representatives from many developed countries argue, or whether this further widens the digital and economic divide.

In 1996, the European Union ratified the Directive on the Legal Protection of Databases, which required countries that were part of the European Union to incorporate this protective legislation within their own national laws. Powerful argumentation continues in favor of strengthening database protection laws that harmonize national legislation with the legislation adopted in the parliament of the European Union. These arguments rest upon the need to protect inventions, patents, and other works in order to encourage private investment in science and the harmonization of legal protection worldwide.[13] These arguments favor more protective legislation that builds upon the concept of sui generis[14] in the protection of databases, resembling the copyright protection of creative works. With its protection of compilation of facts, sui generis represents a considerable threat to worldwide access of large databases, in particular the Human Genome Project.

Following the introduction of the European Union Directive on the Legal Protection of Databases, WIPO was requested to review the need of a worldwide database treaty. In certain sectors in the United States there was strong support for this legislation, even to the extent that it was proposed to increase the original fifteen years proposed by the European Union to twenty-five. Efforts to tighten controls were resisted strongly by the scientific community as well as representatives from the developing world. To provide guidance in formulating government policy in response to the directive and in the context of heated debate, the U.S. National Academy of Science commissioned a study parallel in process to the work that resulted in *The Digital Dilemma*. A Committee for a Study on Promoting Access to Scientific and Technical Data for the Public Interest was formed to identify, review, and make recommendations regarding policy for the protection of private databases while at the same time preserving public access to scientific data in the public interest. The result was a thoughtful report, *A Question of Balance: Private Rights and the Public Interest in Scientific and Technical Databases*.[15] The Committee was well named, as its recommendations demonstrate, for it provides a thoughtful attempt to restore the necessary balance between the private sector and the public good.

A Question of Balance recognizes that the necessary balancing of the interests of database rights holders and the public interest was threatened by these new legal-protection initiatives. The committee concluded that substantial protection of the rights of database owners was already provided under existing legislation and that there was no need for increasing the level of legal protection. There was some scope, however, for developing legislation that would provide an alterative to the more restrictive and controlling regulations put forward by the European Union, and a number of the recommendations in *A Question of Balance* deal with the perceived need to revisit the issue. Certain of these recommendations are particularly relevant to our concerns in this book, as they deal with public access to medical information. One database in particular, GenBank, produced at the U.S. National Center for Biotechnology Information, was built from the direct contributions of scientists around the world. The report recommended that "although private sector databases derived from government data should be eligible for protection, protection should not be extended to databases collected or maintained by the government." It further recommended:

> Limit the term of protection to a period of time sufficient to provide incentive found necessary for the creation of new databases. If legislation with affixed term of protection is adopted an appropriate term of protection most likely should be based on an analysis of the economics of the database industry rather than set arbitrarily.[16]

The centuries-old struggle between competing interests in the battle to preserve the public good is now in the digital arena, and skilled legal arguments have become the basis for the preservation of public interest in the information age.

LIBRARIES AND THEIR ROLE IN THE DEVELOPMENT OF INTELLECTUAL PROPERTY POLICY

Throughout the world librarians are working to comply with copyright law in their individual countries and have been doing so for decades. This may be as straightforward as placing signs on photocopy machines as was done in an earlier era, or it may be through instructing users regarding attribution and fair use rights and responsibilities. Often in today's world, such instruction may include the cautioning of authors regarding signing copyright release forms with publishers. Compliance with existing copyright law is part of daily operations, but some librarians have been courageous in testing the boundaries of publishers' restrictions in the electronic era, particularly as they apply to interlibrary loan and electronic reserve materials, two operations in which electronic journal licenses are particularly restrictive and cumbersome.

At the national level, library associations work in alliance with other organizations to influence legislative developments to guarantee that the enshrined principle of fair use and the balance between the rights of creators and users of copyrighted material is maintained. The international nature of WIPO requires an appropriate library response at an international level, and the International Federation of Library Associations and Institutions (IFLA) has as a priority the balancing of the intellectual property rights of authors with the needs of users. IFLA also maintains a watching brief on economic and trade barriers to the uses of information and developments in the legal arena that impact on libraries. IFLA through its Committee on Copyright and Other Legal Matters (CLM) participates in meetings of WIPO and the World Trade Organization as the voice of library concerns and maintains awareness in the library community of current developments and library interest as these matters evolve.

IFLA's position is determined by its emphasis on universal access, so alliances are naturally with those who support access to information. It has been active in attempting to provoke WIPO into taking a "more balanced and realistic view of the social benefits and costs of intellectual property rights as a tool . . . for supporting creative intellectual activity."[17] IFLA is mindful in its comments of the needs of the developing world in accessing information and advances the recognition that countries that are struggling to meet the basic needs of their people require a different approach to the WIPO copyright compliance. It has drafted an "Access to Knowledge Treaty" (A2K) that enshrines the universal right of access to knowledge and the importance of knowledge for the development of democracy worldwide. If these goals sound familiar, the comments of Stephen Lewis at the beginning of this text are sufficient to emphasize the ongoing nature of the struggle to promote universal access to knowledge. Efforts continue at this point to convince WIPO to incorporate the needs expressed in the A2K Treaty into their policy statements and guidelines. Promoting A2K and the needs of libraries challenges even the most determined librarian advocates as pressure for greater protection of intellectual property and the use of technological protection measures to override fair use proliferate. There is a growing perception in the library and information community that WIPO is overly influenced by the commercial and private sector at the expense of preserving the public domain and the rights of users. The issue is further compounded by the puzzling conclusion by some interest groups that the push for reform within WIPO is based on an antithetical approach to technology.

AN UNCERTAIN FUTURE

The survival of fair use in the digital age as a means to guarantee public interest and access to information is not certain. The thrust and parry of the debates to preserve and enshrine access to information on behalf of those who need it will doubtlessly continue, as they must, for there is much at stake. One of the worrisome issues is in the funding available to some proponents in these debates. Large for-profit corporations that seek to lock up information have the financial resources to engage numerous specialists in intellectual property to lobby and defend their interests. Even when major library associations band together to extend their legal capability to protect the rights of access and availability, they are sadly overwhelmed numerically by lawyers arguing against public access.

The conviction of a number of dedicated librarians worldwide to continue the effort is important and worthy of the respect of the entire library community. If librarians accept the fundamental value and role of providing access to information to all who need to use it, they can assist those worthy few who work with WIPO and national governments worldwide to protect the public interest. In their individual libraries, whether public, medical, or university, they can work to educate their users on the issues of fair use and the economics of information. They can stay informed and articulate on the latest developments in key issues that threaten access to information, and in doing so, can provide a network of strong support that will help to determine whether fair use will survive in the digital age.

NOTES

1. Larry Lessig, *The Future of Ideas: The Fate of the Commons in the Connected World* (New York: Random House, 2001), 20–21.

2. Ronald V. Bettig, *Copyrighting Culture: The Political Economy of Intellectual Property* (New York: Westview Press, 1966), 161.

3. Gary Byrd, "Copyright Compliance in Health Sciences Libraries: A Status Report Two Years after the Implementation of PL94-553," *Bulletin of the Medical Library Association* 69, no. 2 (April 1981): 224–30.

4. U.S. National Academies, *The Digital Dilemma: Intellectual Property in the Information Age* (Washington, DC: National Academy Press, 2000).

5. U.S. National Academies, *The Digital Dilemma*, 69.

6. U.S. National Academies, *The Digital Dilemma*, 205.

7. An Act to Amend the Copyright Act, Assented to April 25, 1997, www.parl.gc.ca/bills/government/C-32/C-32_4/C-32TOCE.html (accessed November 9, 2005).

8. *CCH v. Law Society of Upper Canada*, 2004 SCC 13, www.canlii.org/ca/cas/scc/2004/2004scc13.html (accessed October 5, 2005).

9. An excellent analysis of this case and other aspects of Canadian copyright legislation may be found in Samuel E. Trosow, "The Changing Landscape of Academic Libraries and Copyright Policy: Interlibrary Loans, Electronic Reserves, and Distance Education," in *In the Public Interest: The Future of Canadian Copyright Law*, ed. Michael Geist, 375–407 (Toronto: Irwin Law, 2005).

10. See http://creativecommons.org/about/think (accessed October 6, 2005).

11. A particularly compelling case on the needs of the developing world in this area and an excellent summary of the issues may be found in Martin Khor, *Intellectual Property, Biodiversity and Sustainable Development: Resolving the Difficult Issues* (London: Zed Books, 2002).

12. "A 'Development Agenda' at WIPO: A Shift in IP Policy on the International Stage" (interview with James Love of the Consumer Project on Technology), http://bizlawjournal.ucdavis.edu/article.asp?id=561&print=true (accessed September 30, 2005).

13. The arguments in favor of ratifying the EU directive are summarized in David B. Resnick, "Strengthening the United States' Database Protection Laws: Balancing Public Access and Private Control," *Science and Engineering Ethics* 9, no. 3 (2003): 301–18.

14. 'Sui generis' is a Latin phrase used in legal and philosophical scholarship meaning roughly 'self-made.' To say that something is 'sui generis' means that it stands on its own or is not dependent on other things. A database with sui generic protection has legal protection simply because it is a database: its legal protection does not depend on its status as an original work under copyright law or as an invention under patent law." Resnick, "Strengthening the United States' Database Protection Laws," 303.

15. U.S. National Academy of Sciences, *A Question of Balance: Private Rights and the Public Interest in Scientific and Technical Databases* (Washington, DC: National Research Council, 1999).

16. U.S. National Academy of Sciences, *A Question of Balance*, 1999, http://www.nap.edu/execsumm_pdf/9692.pdf#search (accessed October 16, 2005).

17. IFLANET Committee on Copyright and Other Legal Matters, Report to Council August 2005, Oslo, Norway, http://www.ifla.org/IV/ifla71/clm-councilRep 2005.html (accessed October 18, 2005).

Conclusion

ADVANCING THE ROLE OF THE MEDICAL LIBRARIAN IN THE PUBLIC GOOD

This discussion of medical librarianship over the past one hundred years has provided evidence of the continuing adherence of the profession to a core set of values. Through the exercise of these values medical librarians promote the public good by providing access to medical information for all who need to use it, guaranteeing the continuity of the historical record in the conservation of the documents of medicine and health science, and teaching information literacy. The ways in which these values are expressed have changed beyond recognition over the years since the profession was established by Osler, Charleton, and Gould, but the values have remained constant. However, perennial values are not sufficient to guarantee that the profession endures. To thrive in the twenty-first century, medical librarians must continue in their tradition of adopting the new tools and technologies that evolve to meet the needs of users.

MEDICAL LIBRARIANS IN AN UNCERTAIN FUTURE

Medical librarians are continuing to provide the best possible access to medical information, while facing considerable uncertainty about how medical and scientific information will be provided and preserved in the future. Medical information, both the published literature and the research data on which that literature is based, is now communicated and cataloged in a digital state. Paper, if present at all, is a minor product used in some instances to guarantee the permanence of an archive. This complete conversion has taken place only since the beginning of the twenty-first century.

Today, from the time that they enter school, students learn to search, communicate, and create using the Web and the Internet. This practice is fueled by the ever growing amount of reliable and readily accessible digital content, by broadband extension and hardware and software enhancements, and by online educational opportunities and e-business. But Internet governance and policy have failed to keep pace with these rapid developments in the ways in which society uses information. Policy and legislation is being debated and written retroactively, and different and competing interests are working to influence legislation to support their particular interests. Debates over open access, copyright, and the needs of the consumer and the developing world are all driven by conflicting interest groups and a clash of values regarding policy development.

Due to the importance of medical information in clinical care and in advancing medical research, medical librarians have been at the center of these concerns since the early application of information technology in the 1960s. Medical librarians have developed strong working relationships with publishers and the editorial boards of medical journals, which determine how and what new knowledge will be distributed. We have seen that as early as the 1930s medical librarians reacted against the economics of dramatically increasing costs. Effective as these strategies have been in helping to control the costs of journals, price increases continue at levels that can in many instances not be met. Publishers developed new strategies, and scientific and medical publishing continues to be a lucrative business despite the growth of alternative models in scientific publishing. The global scientific publishing market was estimated at one billion U.S. dollars in 2003, and the International Association of Scientific, Technical and Medical Publishers estimates that there are more than 2,000 STM publishers worldwide, publishing more than 1.2 million articles per year in 16,000 journals.[1]

When the publishing industry first began digital publishing, many libraries became hybrid, with both print and digital journals in one collection. This practice was in fact encouraged by publishers' pricing methods, which priced the digital copy of a journal 10 to 15 percent over the cost of the printed copy. Today, the strategy is totally reversed, as publishers seek to eliminate print versions of their product and users demand online content. In a survey conducted in 2003 by Cox and Cox, 75 percent of the journals published in the United States, Canada, Europe, the United Kingdom, and Asia were available online, with 83 percent of STM titles and 72 percent of humanities and social sciences titles in online versions.[2] The full cast of players—publishers, librarians, users of libraries, and third-party providers such as subscription agents—were dramatically affected by this change. Some, such as subscription agents, were destabilized, and some did not recover. Publishers, who initiated these developments, understand the change best of all and offer many new services to enhance the integrated use of their publications.

As much as information and communications technology has revolutionized medical libraries and the established publishing industry, it has provided even greater opportunity for experimentation and innovation in alternative forms of electronic publishing, for example, the open-access journal. Today, open-access journals represent only a very small part of the scholarly publishing record. Of the 45,091 academic and scholarly titles listed in *Ulrich's Periodical Directory*, 889, or 2 percent, are open-access publications.[3] Despite these figures, open access has emerged in the past few years as a robust alternative to traditional sources that has yet to be fully tested. The journals in the Public Library of Science series have encouraged support for this alternative model. In addition to the creation of new titles published in open access, two innovative parallel developments have emerged: self-archiving and depositing in institutional repositories articles already published in toll-gated journals controlled by commercial publishers. While these developments are being fully tested, there are no clearly preferred alternatives. Subject repositories of publicly available information, in particular the PubMed Central initiative, point the way to new modes of public availability of information while retaining the existing scholarly communication structure. It is not clear which if any of these alternatives will survive or replace the dominant commercial model of research communication. What is clear is that this experimentation is providing creative alternatives in scientific communication and introducing competition into the journal market.

What, then, should the medical librarian be doing? What are the necessary actions that may be taken to determine a future in which medical information is available to all who need to use it regardless of the ability to pay? How can the public be assured that they will be able to read the results of research for which their tax dollars have paid? Supporting alternatives while continuing to provide the best access possible to quality medical information wherever it is published is a reasonable beginning point. However, there are ways in which librarians can be more active and influential.

A MORE ACTIVE APPROACH
TO NEGOTIATIONS WITH PUBLISHERS

Working within the existing institutional and consortial relationships with publishers, there are many improvements that may be achieved through concerted actions by librarians. In the first instance, librarians should work to establish the necessary access to copyrighted literature for all who need to use it. The right of fair use should be the rationale for this access rather than the granting of a minor concession that allows "walk-in use." By the same token, the same level of access should apply to the health care consumer and the patient. The patient who requires medical information should not need to manipulate the existing regulations in a devious manner in order to acquire the information that is essential to recovery. Individuals who are receiving medical care and their families are often already in a vulnerable state due to the threat to health. Further compounding their anxiety through making information inaccessible should not be tolerated.[4] To correct this situation, Librarians need to ensure that the following actions take place.

- The librarian should guarantee that licensed information can be redistributed to a primary user group in an efficient manner. For example, the library should be allowed to distribute to students and faculty electronically copies of journal articles placed on reserve that appear in licensed journals.
- The librarian should guarantee that licensed information may be redistributed electronically for purposes of interlibrary loan.
- The librarian should insist on the right to disclose financial details in any agreement for which the library has signed a license for the output of a publisher.
- The librarian should determine how much the library is willing to pay for information and be prepared not to go beyond a reasonable and agreed-upon ceiling.
- The librarian should exercise sound judgment and return to the principles of collection development by refusing to buy information that is not necessary to the teaching and research programs of the institution, in the spirit of the adage, "If you don't need it, it's not a bargain."[5]

ENSURING THE SURVIVAL OF ALTERNATIVE INITIATIVES IN OPEN-ACCESS PUBLISHING

Alternative publications need the support of the research community if they are to be fairly tested and create the dynamics of change necessary to bring about improved access to information. The medical community, clinicians, and researchers will be the ultimate judges of the value of these new publications. However, it is the medical librarian who must take the initiative of bringing these publications to the attention of the user. In the first instance, the librarian must ensure that these publications are accessible in the same fashion and through the same interface as the established corpus of medical literature. As important as access is, discussion between the librarian and the user is essential to make certain that there is an awareness of these new publications and an assessment of their quality and importance for the development of research and communication. Discussions of the financing of existing dominant publishing models also need to occur to ensure an understanding of why these new initiatives are economically important.

ESTABLISHING INSTITUTIONAL REPOSITORIES

The development of institutional repositories has been greatly assisted by the use of free software, the establishment of metadata standards, and the Open Archives Initiative (OAI), which ensures the exchange of electronic information. However part of the work of the librarian must be the nurturing of these repositories by encouraging faculty to deposit their publications in them. The assistance of faculty is an absolutely essential component of these repositories' success. To enlist faculty collaboration requires that the faculty member have support for modifying their copyright agreements with publishers to enable this deposit and that the actual deposit be simple and not consume any significant fraction of the author's time. There are no technical barriers to the establishment of institutional repositories. But where they exist, they are not growing at a substantial rate. The research community needs to be convinced that this is an exercise that is worth the effort.

One of the most successful models of the development of repositories on a national scale is the DARE project in the Netherlands,[6] a national system of institutional repositories that invites only the top two hundred researchers to deposit their publications in repositories in a project known as "The Cream of Science." Approximately 60 percent of the articles are fully available, with the remaining blocked by copyright. Clearly, there is added value to the researchers in having their publications considered eligible, and the prestige factor is well addressed in the conceptualization of this initiative. This program was launched at a conference jointly hosted by the SURF Foundation of the Netherlands, Britain's Joint Information Systems

Committee (JISC), and the Coalition for Networked Information (CNI) in Amsterdam in May 2005. The SURF Foundation is active in studying the development of institutional repositories in Europe, North America, and Australia and in encouraging the development of these initiatives.[7]

MEDICAL LIBRARIANS AND THE PROMOTION OF HEALTH THROUGH CLINICAL AND PATIENT INFORMATION

Many of the above-mentioned actions for the improvement of access to medical information impact on the availability of such information to the general public. We have seen in the chapters on improving access to information for patients, health care professionals, and the general public that medical librarians have maintained creative and active approaches to the distribution of information to these constituencies. Both in the print and digital eras, medical librarians have recognized that the important point was the delivery of the necessary information when and where it was needed. The development of the concept of the clinical medical librarian, the idea of the informationist, and the Grateful Med program of the U.S. National Library of Medicine all emphasized the delivery of highly specific and current clinical information efficiently extracted from the sea of medical knowledge.

A number of commercial publishers' initiatives have also recognized the importance of delivering precise medical information to the point of need. They have been successful in "unbundling" and "rebundling" comprehensive packages of journals produced by a particular publisher and have licensed the rights to include selected titles in new packages of medical information focused around medical specialties. These electronic resources are subscription based and include frequent updates as well as other information such as practice guidelines, and they often emphasize evidenced-based medicine. They provide busy clinicians with all the information that they think they need. Yet most of this information is already available in the large packages of journals licensed by the library! As a result of the repackaging, the catalog of the holdings of a particular library may list three or four copies of the same journal, representing the different licenses to journal packages to which the medical library subscribes.

This situation leads to the suspicion that medical librarians have not yet been able to develop ways of delivering highly specialized services in a comprehensive manner. If they had, these new services would probably not have found a market, at least among health professionals who had access to a reasonably resourced medical library. The reason this has not happened is that medical librarians are not typically sufficiently well funded to develop these specialized services and to integrate them into the ongoing programs of the library. Such focused information services require both time and talent in their development and may not be sustainable without ongoing financial support.

Both these needs—to improve the medical information available to the clinician in the process of treating the patient and to improve the patient's understanding of illness and treatment—converge in the interaction of the individual physician and patient. The patient's need for and right to information are further strengthened by the legal requirement of informed choice. It is surprising to find that medical librarians are not always thought of at an early stage in filling the information needs of both the physician and the patient.

A recent article on the improvement of patient information and the role of physicians, nurses, and other health care professionals proposes solutions to the improvement of informed choice.[8] Possible sources of patient information were clinicians, who may or may not be knowledgeable in informed-choice counseling, and the possibility of training other health professionals as "impartial decision counselors." One possible solution to the improvement of patient information that is proposed is the inclusion of informed-choice counseling in the education of doctors and nurses. The preferred option is the training of third-party decision counselors. Although these decision counselors are not medical experts, they would function as "highly skilled knowledge brokers." The offices of these decision counselors would be located in a quiet environment, provide high-speed Internet access on workstations, and include a complete library of decision aids and other education materials. Further, these counselors would be located in offices conveniently accessible to hospitals and outpatient services, suitable to serving individual practitioners. Although the article includes reference to the work of Davidoff and Florance[9] on the development of the informationist (see chapter 8 on clinical information), the potential of building on the existing hospital library and its medical librarian is notable by its absence.

What can the medical librarian conclude from this article? Clearly, the services that the library is currently providing are not fully recognized. Further, there is an emerging and recognized need for highly skilled knowledge workers to extract, analyze, and discuss patient information. It is equally clear in the Woolf article that librarians are not perceived as possible providers of this information and, therefore, not perceived as possessing the requisite skills. It is incumbent on the medical library profession to identify the necessary knowledge and skills that are required to fill this need and to recruit into the profession of medical librarianship those individuals who possess the potential to fill this role. At the same time, it is likely that some currently practicing medical librarians do rise to this need. In a profession that developed the technical and medical literacy necessary to support access to medical information, this new challenge does not appear to be insurmountable.

MEDICAL LIBRARIANS AND THE PRESERVATION OF THE HISTORY OF THE HEALTH SCIENCES

Preserving the accumulated medical knowledge of the past is one of the core values of the profession of medical librarianship, although it may not have received the attention that has been given to the providing of access to medical information. There are a number of reasons for this, not the least of which is the fact that many hospital and medical libraries are not mandated to provide and preserve information that is not of current value. They are able to rely upon other institutions to preserve the documents of the medical past. It would not be consistent or realistic to expect libraries that are focused exclusively on current medical information to do otherwise. We have explored earlier in this book the crucial role played by the U.S. National Library of Medicine in providing a comprehensive and reliable plan for the preservation and conservation of the history of medicine. But the functions of a professional librarian are not defined solely by the place of work. The values of the profession encourage all medical librarians to be knowledgeable about preservation practices as they relate to the medical literature, to make sound decisions regarding the materials in the collections for which they are responsible, and to influence and support the development of local and national preservation strategies.

Recently a most revealing exchange of comments took place on a listserv for medical librarians concerning a problem with the completeness of a particular journal article in digital form.[10] The story is interesting as it also relates to the practice referred to as the bundling of the same journal in several journal packages. In attempting to locate a complete copy of a particular journal article, the medical librarian discovered that the library held a number of copies of the journal in electronic form. Nevertheless, a complete copy of the article could not be located. This discovery was followed by the inference that the library should think carefully before canceling print subscriptions in order to avoid such problems. This conclusion cannot be justified. The move toward digital-only medical and scientific journals is rapid, inexorable, and justified. The problem was not the fact that the journal was in digital form; it was in the failure to maintain high standards in the production of a digital version. As librarians make decisions to license journals in electronic form, they need to build in certain guarantees and penalty clauses if the material for which they are paying is flawed. In any commercial transaction the return of flawed merchandise is allowed. For some time librarians have been drawing problems of errors and incompleteness to the attention of the publisher. It seems reasonable to include a guarantee of quality in licenses to ensure that the necessary care will be taken during the production stage. The problem is a human problem, not a technical one.

Guaranteeing continuing access in perpetuity to electronic journals is a matter of increasingly urgent concern to all librarians. The history of science and medicine from the nineteenth century to the present is told in large measure through the journal literature. Thus the preservation of an increasingly digital history becomes imperative to the historical record of medical and scientific research. Yet continuing access is threatened. Librarians need to take responsibility to ensure the necessary survival of the historical record. In the paper era, there existed a large amount of redundancy in copies of journals, which resulted from the numerous subscriptions to paper journals in a number of libraries. This provided some guarantee that at least one copy would survive. National Libraries such as the U.S. National Library of Medicine and the British Library and large research libraries such as the Countway Library at Harvard or the Library of the Wellcome Trust in London would formally take responsibility for preservation.

But the digital revolution and the electronic journal changed this model. No longer did duplicate copies exist. One copy of an electronic journal housed on the publisher's server was all that was necessary to serve multiple license holders worldwide. Preservation in this world faces not one but two challenges: the preservation of documents that were born digital, such as e-journals, and the conversion of existing print to digital format, which has become increasingly important as the research community has adapted to electronic journals. While it may not be true that the printed science journal is dead, it is not an exaggeration to say that it is deeply buried! Librarians are just at the beginning of finding effective solutions and guarantees to ensure the survival of the digital historical record. The half-life of appropriate technologies is one major issue; preservation of digital documents requires the migration of data as technologies change. Medical librarians will find strong partners and vigorous leadership in working to preserve e-journals. The well-developed JSTOR program[11] is an initiative that has demonstrated the possibility of reliable, high-quality journal digitization that converts print to digital format. There is a wealth of research available through the foundation studies on digital preservation done by the Council on Library and Information Resources.[12]

Today at many universities, digitization laboratories exist with various degrees of capability. It is important that medical librarians with rich historical collections have access to or develop the capability to digitize materials. Indeed, the preservation of an original copy is better guaranteed when a digital surrogate is available to provide the required access to content. And that content can be delivered anywhere that it is required. In developing a strategy for preservation, librarians need to consider the policies and practices of other libraries and the role of the publisher. They need to work collaboratively in developing tools and facilities, as these are costly and in more than one instance lie unused a large part of the time. Librarians need to be aware of what is happening in the practices of preservation of both print and electronic documents. They also need to be alert to rare and unique materials that may exist in their own local environment and work to ensure that this material is preserved and available.

EPILOGUE

This review of the history and development of the profession of medical librarianship has served to strengthen understanding of the three core values of medical librarianship and to demonstrate how these values evolved in a changing environment over the course of more than a century. With the arrival of the Internet and a new era of information technology and communication, change occurred in every aspect of the work of medical libraries, but these values persisted.

The distinctive and substantial contribution of medical librarians to the advancement of librarianship in general has also been a part of this story. As early adopters of technology, leaders in insisting on the needs of the public, and determined providers of excellence in service who were ready to address the problems and costs of scholarly communication and to continuously upgrade their professional skills, medical librarians may justifiably look at their role and their profession with pride.

It is clear that future challenges are profound. These challenges will best be met through greater collaboration between librarians working in all facets of librarianship. At the same time as they work to advance their special field, medical librarians will need to look to colleagues in university and public libraries. Their collaboration on the challenges of public access, information literacy, and preservation of heritage materials is essential. New partnerships with funding agencies, foundations and publishers, and researchers and clinicians will help to achieve the goals of all concerned. What is required is a collective intelligence to address the magnitude of the challenge that lies ahead.

NOTES

1. Organisation for Economic Co-operation and Development, *Digital Broadband Content: Scientific Publishing* (Paris: OECD, 2005), 106. This thoughtful recent study provides a useful quantitative analysis of contemporary scientific publishing and evaluates objectively the advantages and disadvantages of recent developments such as the Big Deal and new models of scientific publishing that are emerging in the digital age.

2. Quoted in OECD, *Digital Broadband Content*, 46.

3. OECD, *Digital Broadband Content*, 62.

4. A particularly dramatic case is the one experienced by Sharon Terry. Terry, the mother of children suffering from pseudoxanthoma elasticum (PXE), a genetic disease that is rare and without a known cure, faced great difficulty in obtaining the "locked-up" scientific information that deals with the disease. She describes the convoluted ways she had to develop in order to access this necessary information, which had been published in journals that were under license. In the process of struggling with this information deficit she discovered the Alliance for Tax Payer Access, a group working to support public access to research funded by taxpayers. She is currently president of the Genetic Alliance, which is part of the Alliance for Taxpayer Access. Her experiences are described in Sharon Terry, "In the Public Interest: Open Access," *College and Research Libraries News* 66, no. 7 (July–August 2005), available at http://www.ala.org/ala/acrl/acrlpubs/crlnews/backissues2005/julyaugust05/publicinterest.html (accessed December 16, 2005).

5. Several of these proposals were developed during a working group of an invitational meeting held at Cornell University, October 9–11, 2005, The Janus Conference on Research Library Collections: Managing the Shifting Ground between Writers and Readers.

6. DARE Digital Academic Repositories: Een SURF Programma, http://www.creamofscience.org (accessed December 15, 2005).

7. Gerard van Westrienen and Clifford A. Lynch, "Academic Institutional Repositories," *D-Lib Magazine* 11, no. 9 (September 2005), http://www.dlib.org/dlib.html (accessed July 14, 2006).

8. Steven H. Woolf et al., "Promoting Informed Choice: Transforming Health Care to Dispense Knowledge for Decision Making," *Annals of Internal Medicine* 143, no. 4 (August 16, 2005): 293–300.

9. Frank Davidoff and Valerie Florance, "The Informationist: A New Health Profession?" [editorial], *Annals of Internal Medicine* 132, no. 12 (June 20, 2000): 996–98.

10. MEDLIB-L@LISTSERV.Buffalo.edu (posted October 25, 2005).

11. For a full description see http://www.jstor.org/about/desc.html (accessed October 31, 2005). This Andrew W. Mellon–funded program is not a current database but provides complete runs of backfiles. It includes some general science, mathematics and statistics, and ecology and botany journals. The project is well recognized by the care it took in converting the paper versions to digital form in completeness and comprehensiveness. It provides a useful model of high-quality digitization.

12. For a description of the work of this organization and a list of their publications that are available over the Internet see http://www.clir.org/pubs/reports/reports.html (accessed October 31, 2005).

BIBLIOGRAPHY

This bibliography includes only monographs that have been consulted in the writing of this book. The endnotes to the chapters contain numerous citations to journal articles that were consulted in both print and electronic form. The journals that were most heavily used included the *Journal of the Medical Library Association*, *Health Libraries Review*, *Library Trends* (for special theme issues on medical libraries), *Bibliotheca Medica Canadiana*, and the *Newsletters* of the Association of Research Libraries and the Council on Library and Information Resources. The websites of numerous organizations—Scholarly Publishing and Academic Research Coalition (SPARC), the Dutch Higher Education and Research Partnership (SURF) and Digital Academic Repositories (DARE), the Association of Research Libraries (ARL), the Canadian Association of Research Libraries (CARL), and the International Federation of Library Associations and Institutions (IFLA)—were also of great help.

Adams, Scott. *Medical Bibliography in an Age of Discontinuity*. Chicago: Medical Library Association, 1981.

Baker, Nicholson. *Double Fold: Libraries and the Assault on Paper*. New York: Random House, 2001.

Bettig, Ronald V. *Copyrighting Culture: The Political Economy of Intellectual Property*. New York: Westview Press, 1996.

Brodman, Estelle. *The Development of Medical Bibliography*. Chicago: Medical Library Association, 1954.

Bunting, Alison. *The Nation's Health Information Network: History of the Regional Medical Library Program, 1965–1985*. Chicago: Medical Library Association, 1987.

Connor, Jennifer. *Guardians of Medical Knowledge: The Genesis of the Medical Library Association*. Lanham, MD: Medical Library Association and Scarecrow Press, 2000.

Diodato, Virgil. *The Dictionary of Bibliometrics*. New York: Haworth Press, 1994.

Donohue, Joseph C. *Understanding Scientific Literatures: A Bibliometric Approach*. Cambridge, MA: MIT Press, 1973.

Garvey, William D. *Communication: The Essence of Science*. Oxford: Pergamon Press, 1979.

Geist, Michael, ed. *In the Public Interest: The Future of Canadian Copyright Law*. Toronto: Irwin Law, 2005.

Gorman, Michael. *Our Enduring Values: Librarianship in the 21st Century*. Chicago: American Library Association, 2000.

Guédon, Jean-Claude. *In Oldenburg's Long Shadow—Librarians, Research Scientists, Publishers and the Control of Scientific Publishing*. Washington, DC: Association of Research Libraries, 2001.

Hirsch, E. D. *Cultural Literacy: What Every American Needs to Know*. Boston: Houghton Mifflin, 1987.

Holly, Edward G. *Raking the Historic Coals*. Chicago, Beta Phi Mu, 1967.

Horton, Richard. *Health Wars: On the Global Front Lines of Modern Medicine*. New York: New York Review of Books, 2004.

Information on Disease Management and Therapy: Issues and Options for the Canadian Health Network: December 15, 2003. Montreal: James Henderson and Associates, 2003.

Kaul, Inge, ed. *Providing Global Public Goods: Managing Globalization*. Published for the United Nations Development Programme. New York: Oxford University Press, 2003.

Khor, Martin. *Intellectual Property, Biodiversity and Sustainable Development: Resolving the Difficult Issues*. London: Zed Books, 2002.

Kronick, David A. *A History of Scientific and Technical Periodicals*, 2d ed. Metuchen, N.J.: Scarecrow Press, 1976.

Kyrillidou, Martha, and Mark Young, comp. and ed. *ARL Statistics, 2002—2003: A Compilation of Statistics from the One Hundred and Twenty-Three Members of the Association of Research Libraries*. Washington, DC: Association of Research Libraries, 2004.

Lessig, Larry. *The Future of Ideas: The Fate of the Commons in the Connected World*. New York: Random House, 2001.

Licklider, J. C. R. *Libraries of the Future*. Cambridge, MA: MIT Press, 1965.

Meadows, A. J. ed. *Development of Science Publishing in Europe*. Amsterdam: Elsevier Science, 1980.

Merton, Robert K. *The Sociology of Science: Theoretical and Empirical Investigations*. Chicago: University of Chicago Press, 1973.

Miles, Wyndham D. *A History of the National Library of Medicine, the Nation's Treasury of Medical Knowledge* (NIH Publication No. 82-1904). Washington, DC: U.S. Public Health Service, National Institutes of Health, National Library of Medicine, 1982.

Moschovitis, Christos J. P., Hillary Poole, Tami Schuyler, and Theresa M. Senft. *History of the Internet: A Chronology, 1843 to the Present*. Santa Barbara, CA: ABC-CLIO, 1999.

Price, Derek J. de Solla. *Little Science, Big Science*. New York: Columbia University Press, 1963.

Rees, Alan M. *Consumer Health Information Source Book*, 6th ed. Phoenix, AZ: Oryx Press, 2000.

———. *Consumer Health Information Source Book*, 7th ed. Phoenix, AZ: Oryx Press, 2003.

Simon, Beatrice. *Library Support of Medical Education and Research in Canada*. Ottawa: Association of Canadian Medical Colleges, 1964.

Starr, Paul. *The Social Transformation of American Medicine*. New York: Basic Books, 1982.

———. *The Creation of the Media: The Political Origins of Modern Communications*. New York: Basic Books, 2004.

INDEX

ABOUT THE AUTHOR

Frances K. Groen received undergraduate and library science degrees from the University of Toronto. She holds a master's degree in the history and philosophy of science from the University of Pittsburgh. She has held professional appointments at the University of Toronto, Stanford University, the University of Pittsburgh, and McGill University. She served as curator of the history of medicine at the Falk Library of the Health Professions, University of Pittsburgh, and for eighteen years headed McGill University's medical library. She was the founding Trenholme Director of Libraries at McGill and is now emeritus director. In 1983 she was a senior fellow at the University of California at Los Angeles. She has served on numerous boards, including the Association of Research Libraries, the Center for Research Libraries, and the International Federation of Library Associations and Institutions. She was elected to the presidencies of the Medical Library Association (1989–1990) and the Canadian Association of Research Libraries (1999–2001). In 1997, she was appointed a fellow of the Medical Library Association. She was named the Canadian Association of College and University Librarians' Outstanding Academic Librarian in 1996 and received the Canadian Association of Research Libraries Award for Distinguished Service to Research Librarianship in 2004. She is the author of more than forty journal articles that have appeared in the *Journal of the Medical Library Association, College and Research Libraries, Bibliotheca Medica Canadiana, Library Resources and Technical Services*, and *Health Libraries Review*. Her home is in Montreal, where she lives with her husband, Jean-Claude Guédon.